real
Gorgeous

real Gorgeous

The truth about body and beauty

KAZ COOKE

BLOOMSBURY

Cover: *Our radiant covergirl, Hermoine the Modern Girl, is wearing a frock from a Chiswick jumble sale. Hair by accident. Styling: hardly likely. Make-up: old lipstick from the bottom of her handbag from which the label has worn off. There may have been eyebrow pencil involvement, although this is by no means certain. Shoes: model's own. Underpants: yes. Signature fragrance: Eau de Faff, by Serge-Penelope Froufrou de Prohibitively Expensif. Photographed exclusively for* Real Gorgeous *by the Mervyn Purvis Agency, Paris, Rome, New York, Moscow and Llandrindod Wells. All rights reserved.*

89464
646.7 coo

The author and publisher of this book cannot be held liable for any errors and omissions, or actions that may be taken as a consequence of using it.

All rights reserved; no part of this publication may be reproduced, stored in a retrieval system, or transmitted by any means, electronic, mechanical, photocopying or otherwise, without the prior permission of the Publisher.

First published in 1994

This paperback edition first published 1996

First published in Britain 1995 by Bloomsbury Publishing Plc, 2 Soho Square, London W1V 6HB

Copyright © text and cartoons 1995 by Kaz Cooke

The moral right of the author has been asserted

British Library Cataloguing in Publication Data

A CIP record for this book is available from the British Library

ISBN 0 7475 2696 6

10 9 8 7 6 5 4 3 2 1

Cover concept by Julia Church and Lin Tobias
Cover illustrations by Kaz Cooke
Text design by text-art
Typeset by Hewer Text Composition Services, Edinburgh
Printed in Britain by Cox & Wyman Ltd, Reading

Contents

Acknowledgements

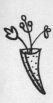

Chris ('of all the places I've been, libraries are the sexiest') Pip was the researcher on *Real Gorgeous*: my thanks to her for panting amongst the shelves, the interviews with research subjects, and her efficient collating and presentation of the right stuff. The British edition was edited by Kate Bouverie.

For supplying, interpreting and checking information, thanks are due to Penelope Goward, the Australasian College of Dermatologists and its swag of helpful experts, Dr Neil Hewson, Sue Noy, The Alcohol and Drug Foundation, the Anorexia and Bulimia Association of Victoria, the Royal Prince Alfred Hospital Eating Disorders Clinic, Rosemary Stanton, Ruth Trickey and Penelope Tree.

Thank you also to the staff of the *Age* newspaper library in Melbourne and the Condé Nast library in New York, to the students who copied the graffiti on college and university toilet walls about body image in response to my letter published in campus newspapers, and to the editors of *Dolly* and *Cleo* magazines for printing my request for letters about body image.

I am particularly grateful to all the women who wrote to me with their thoughts on many related issues. Each was useful. Excerpts from these letters appear as edited quotes throughout the book. All names have been changed, and some locations have been shuffled.

The cartoons on pages 157, 159 and 161 also feature on Roland Harvey greeting cards.

Cynthia Heimel quotes from *Get Your Tongue out of My Mouth, I'm Kissing You Goodbye* (Picador, London, 1993). Victoria Wood quotes from *Mens Sana In Thingummy Doodah* (Mandarin, London, 1993) and *Up to You Porky* (Mandarin, London, 1993). Extract from the BBC programme 'French and Saunders' reproduced with the permission of Dawn French, Jennifer Saunders and the BBC.

Extract from 'Magazine' episode reproduced from *Absolutely Fabulous* with the permission of Jennifer Saunders and BBC Enterprises Limited.

The book you hold was culled from a wee mountain of information, with a great deal of help and support. Thank you Chris Pip, Julie Gibbs, Anna Dollard, Jenna Mead, Mary Sinclair, Sharon Connolly, Mark Davis, Foong Ling Kong, Glenda Jones, Philippa Hawker and Lisby Gore.

Introduction

We need something that will cheer up anybody who has 'the uglies'. Something to reassure all certifiably gorgeous girls and women that they are not Space Porkers from Hell.

We need the facts which will make us RELAX, not the over-wrought opinions that send us fleeing to stupid diets, insane over-exercising and mirror-misery. We want to find out how to stop seeing our bodies as the enemy. And hey, let's face it, we wouldn't mind a laugh while we're at it.

We need some help with self-esteem which cuts through the mixed messages of magazine articles called 'Love your own body' illustrated only by professionally-lit, re-touched photos of a size-8, six-foot-tall, 13-year-old aerobics instructor-model wearing a frilly baby-doll dress, platform thigh-boots and a terminally bored expression.

We need to get away from too many dry statistics, relentless academic essays, incomprehensible diagrams and scientific formulas that don't seem to relate to real life. We need stuff which frees us to make up our own minds. And maybe cartoons would be a lot more fun than endless pictures of models.

We need a book that isn't just about theory but about action: *how* to break out of the useless dieting cycle, *how* to deal with dorks who make comments about our appearance, *how* to accept a natural womanly shape, whether tall, small, thin or rounded.

We'd like to know how to avoid and deal with eating disorders, and what we can eat without panicking. We want the truth about skincare products: which cheap ones work and which ones advertise using pretend science, fancy French and straight-out lies. We want to have fun with clothes and make-up, not feel that we have to spend a fortune on stuff to blindly follow fashion.

We need to know why cosmetic surgery is not about simple 'nips and tucks', but pain, and gouging, and self-hatred and desperation that has other answers than the knife. We'd like to be able to laugh off the *Allure* magazine suggestion that face-lift bandages might become 'a fashion trend'.

We need some information that, unlike magazines, isn't influenced by advertising. A book that isn't trying to sell you anything except more self-confidence and the truth. Something that we can always open to remind ourselves that it's okay that we have different shapes, different sizes and different skin. (Not to mention the odd tuft of body hair.) A book that we can run to any time we feel like screaming at the very sight of a cakie thing.

In short, we need a book that gathers all this stuff together, combines the facts and the fun and gives us some options about where to look for more help if we need it.

I couldn't find such a book, so I had to write one. Here it is.

Kaz Cooke

real
Gorgeous

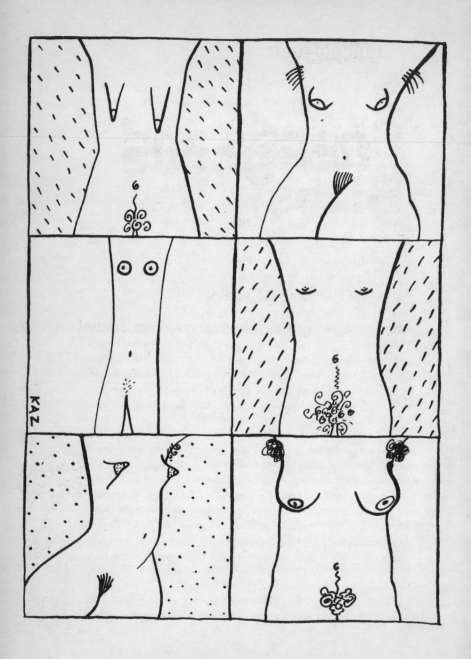

chapter one

Shapes and Sizes

In the beginning

Whoopsie, where did these curvy bits come from? Like a little old caterpillar programmed to become a butterfly, our grown-up shapes are already decided before we are born. When we get to puberty, we find out what kind of a butterfly we are.

The teenage years: who needs 'em? Is the world deliberately trying to confuse us or what? We're sitting around minding our own business and suddenly our bodies go *berserk*.

Our shape changes dramatically, we grow to our full height, start periods, gain extra breast tissue and other fat deposits in our lower body. (It lasts from about age ten until about 15, although the changes sometimes don't finish until your early twenties.)

There's the arrival of hair in previously bald places. Very often 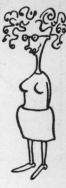 one breast grows larger than the other for some time until the other one catches up, but the right one often ends up slightly larger. Vaginal lips enlarge. There's extra sweating.

Everyone gets terribly embarrassed and wants to hide their bits. Nobody feels much like a beautiful butterfly. Sometimes it feels more like being a squished caterpillar.

In many other cultures these rites of passage are celebrated with ceremony, which would seem a more healthy way of going about it.

This is the sort of time any reasonable society would send its children on a long holiday, complete with instructions on how to be an adult and why you're still gorgeous. Instead they give you exams. Weird.

The changes happen differently for each person, at different speeds. Sometimes, people go BOING. On average, girls start their changes two or three years before boys. Hormonal changes often induce pimples as well (thank you so much, I think I'd rather just have the hips). Girls will put on one and a half to two and a half stone during this time and grow to maximum height with a few more pounds to come before they turn 20 or so.

Before puberty, girls have 10 to 15 per cent more fat than boys. After puberty, they have 20 to 30 per cent more fat than boys. Both sexes have a growth spurt, the male one being mostly in muscle and lean tissue, the female in fat tissue.

Anyway, the point is, we put on more flesh on our hips while boys lose it. Suddenly – oh my GOD – you think you're getting fat. You're getting bigger in all the areas you've heard women complain about and loathe and pinch with rueful expressions. But you're not get-

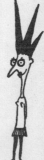

ting fat at all. You're becoming a woman. The much-criticised pear shape is natural. When girls become women, fat is deposited around their hips and stomach in preparation for fertility and protection for the uterus, should you decide to avail yourself of its possibilities.

Breasts are also made up mostly of fat tissue. The extent of these changes are governed by genetics. (You may be told you have your auntie's breasts, and wonder if you should give them back.) Your

> Being thin ain't all it's cracked up to be. I'm 18, five feet four, just over seven stone and size eight. I'm a very light frame and I'm one of those people who can eat bucketloads of food and not put on an ounce. It's almost impossible to get clothes that fit properly. Get sick, and forget it, I soon resemble a skeleton, my hipbones protrude, as well as every other bone it seems. It's really scary to lose three-quarters of a stone when you're already thin. It does get embarrassing to hear all those girls with what I consider perfectly healthy, gorgeous bodies envying my figure. I never see their size, I see past their body shape to look at what's inside them. It's our minds that make our bodies either embarrassing or acceptable. I've had so many guys comment on the fact that it's nice to see a girl enjoy her food.
>
> Kimberley, 18

eventual shape, programmed into you before you were born, may be a different cocktail of genes from your brothers or sisters.

Girls who mature early may be shorter, heavier for their height and

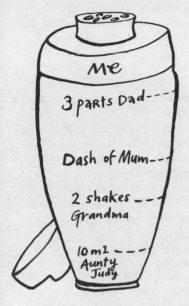

have shorter legs than girls who mature later. These girls are hit with a double whammy of feeling changed and different before their thinner, taller friends, and also less like the thin ideal they may feel they have to conform to. Others may be 'late bloomers'.

Even girls with small breasts and slight hips go through the changes. They are no less women for having fewer curves. Their bodies, too, have made the necessary changes during puberty.

Some adolescent girls delay these changes by exercising too much and underfeeding themselves. Their body shapes are retarded at an earlier growth stage and the onset of periods delayed. This is common in ballet and gymnastics students and

athletes, and shamefully encouraged by some teachers. One study showed ballet dancers delayed the onset of menstruation for an average of three years.

One hundred years ago the average age to begin menstruation in the well-fed parts of the world was sixteen. It's now between twelve-and-a-half and thirteen. This is thought to be due to improved nutrition, or possibly Mars Bars.

You can't change your shape By the time you've been through puberty, you'll know whether you're going to be tall and thin or tall and big or short and curvy. What about all those people who say you can change your shape through diet and exercise? Not true: you can change your weight overall but not the general pattern

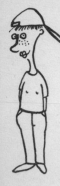

of weight distribution. What's more, your distribution of fat and muscle fibre were also programmed into you before you were born.

Fat patterns differ between people, but they are not changed by dieting. Most women who diet regain their previous body weight within a year (more on this in the diet section), and the body will return to its natural shape after excessive exercising and dieting are stopped.

In another study 'Is Body Fat Distribution Changed by Dieting?' John Garrow concluded that, 'With weight loss the waist–hip ratio does not change but the waist–thigh ratio decreases. This is to be expected since in obesity there is a relatively greater deposit of fat on the waist than on the thighs' (e.g. a big beer belly).

What the man is trying to say in doctorspeak is that there is no proof that more fat is lost from one body part and not others during weight loss. In

> My body is pear-shaped and I can't stand it, my hips and thighs are way too big for what I want. I've tried many different diets but can never seem to stick to them. I always end up pigging out on junk food then I feel guilty and don't eat for two or three days, hoping to lose the weight I put on. I read this can be bad for you but that doesn't bother me, I just want to lose weight.
>
> Anonymous

other words, you're still going to be the same shape after dieting – just lighter. And you'll still be the same shape after exercising – only leaner.

Another study showed that physical training may not reduce body weight (as muscle replaces fat) but could reduce the waist–hip ratio by between 3 and 6 per cent: nowhere near enough to be noticeable to the naked eye. The study found that fat cells on the bottom, hips and thighs were more difficult to reduce than the abdominal fat cells.

The fat controllers Dr Sandra Cabot, Australian author of *The Body Shaping Diet,* claims that there are four body types. Android (strong, thickset, relatively uncurvy, more 'masculine', extra fat deposited above the pelvis); gynaeoid (the majority: pear-shaped, extra fat deposited on the thighs, buttocks, breasts and later the lower abdomen); lymphatic (generalised thickening and puffiness due to fluid retention especially in the limbs and fat distribution all over the body. 'Lymphatic women have often been "chubby" since childhood', says Dr Cabot); and thyroid (narrow, long-limbed, smaller-breasted with weight gain occurring first around the abdomen and upper thighs).

The problem with this sort of theory is that there are not only four different body types. There are millions, all bodies with different metabolisms, genes, environments, colouring, ways of life, culturally determined and geographically determined eating habits, all with different hormonal influences, ages, places in the cycle of life and times in the menstrual cycle.

Like many people living in confusing times, Dr Cabot speaks of control. 'Women want knowledge about how they can help themselves so they can get a feeling of control in their lives.' It is dangerous to equate control over your life with impossible control over your body shape. Who has control over everything anyway? (And can they be stopped?!)

The Body Shaping Diet, like other books claiming to change the shape of one part of the body (*The Hip and Thigh Diet* and others), sells by claiming to be a 'breakthrough in weight control'. Dr Cabot claims that the diets will get rid of cellulite. 'Cellulite is unsightly', she told *Who Weekly*, which ran a cover story on her theories. 'But if it doesn't concern you, don't worry about it.' How encouraging.

She concludes, '[My] book is about giving women the chance of

> Now that I'm a mum I'm especially interested in mothers' figures. I look at all Demi Moore's semi-nude shots to see if she had stretch marks and a flabby stomach. And with her *Vanity Fair* cover, why didn't I look like that when I was pregnant with my second child?
>
> Annie, 24
>
> *Because you didn't have full body make-up, professional lighting, a day-long team of make-up and hair artists, and airbrushing and retouching of the photographs before publication. Because you don't have a team of housekeepers and nannies so you can do three to seven boring hours of gym work a day, as Demi Moore said she did following the birth of each child. Like other actresses, she has body doubles available to her for close-ups if she chooses.*

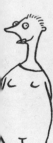

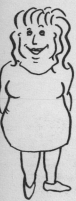

getting off their bums and eating the right food'. One gets the impression that Dr Cabot is dead against women sitting on their bums: 'I am a woman who controls her life completely'. Dr Cabot admitted to being about half a stone underweight, 'so busy I don't eat properly'. Her co-author, a naturopath, said, 'whenever we travel together I make sure we have breakfast and dinner'.

Dr Cabot has not convinced others in the medical profession that special foods in combinations will target fat on one area of the body. She concedes that body type is genetically coded but insists, 'You can lose weight in specific areas just by having the right food combinations to balance your metabolism'. Her diets, for example, ban dairy foods for lymphatic (large) women and stimulants for thyroid (thin) women.

Her description of thyroid-shaped women as 'the envy of all others', inclined to be 'highly strung' and 'prone to eating disorders like anorexia' prompted many of *Who Weekly*'s readers to write and complain that they were tall and thin, not highly strung, and certainly not prone to eating disorders. Dr Cabot had suggested that the Princess of Wales's body shape rather than her state of mind was characteristic of bulimics.

Despite the hopes of women who read this kind of stuff, full control over your life is an impossible enough goal without expecting that you can control your hip shape as well.

Recently Australian *Cosmopolitan* ran a full-page photograph of model Naomi Campbell with the screaming headline: 'Is this the Perfect Body?' and answered: 'Yes it probably is – the perfect combination of strength and femininity. This body belongs to supermodel Naomi Campbell but you, too, can achieve Naomi's fit, shapely look.'

The magazine went on to describe 'the body' – not the woman but the packaging – as '175 cm (5ft 8) of absolute perfection. Twenty-one-year-old Naomi's body is a work of art. Her well-defined, wide shoulders and 86-cm (34-in) bust taper down to a 58-cm (23-in) waist and slim 86-cm (34-in) hips, with a pert bottom and long, shapely legs.' This erotic description was next to a picture of an oiled Naomi Campbell almost in the nude (in high heels and holding a length of shiny, red fabric) with her back to the camera and looking back over her shoulder.

'For Naomi, a superb body was a gift of nature – for the rest of us it is something that can be attained with a good diet, exercise, willpower and determination.' The magazine noted that Ms Campbell weighed only 48 kilograms (seven and a half stone), with body fat of about 16 per cent, almost certainly too low for regular periods, if any at all. It reported that 16 per cent was 'just over half that of an average Australian woman's count of 30 per cent on a typical 63-kilogram (nine stone nine), 160-cm (5ft 3) frame'.

Cosmo's editor began a subsequent magazine with an apology. 'Whoops did we ever get it wrong! But we're not guilty of irresponsibility as some of our readers suggested. What we are guilty of is inaccuracy. Our story put the beautiful black English model's weight at 48 kilos. When your letters began to arrive we contacted Naomi's agent and found that she in fact weighs in at around 54.5 kilos (about eight and a half stone).'

'As the editor of a magazine that has the glamour image *Cosmo* has,' continued editor Pat Ingram, 'I'm often accused of promoting an unrealistic beauty ideal. I don't believe this is true. Certainly our fashion and beauty pages feature good-looking, slim models, but they are just that, models – girls who make their living from their looks, girls who conform to society's current standards of physical female beauty. Ideally, every woman would be slim: it not only looks better, it's healthier. It's when the pursuit of *slim* becomes the obsession to be *thin* that the danger sets in' (her emphases).

Slim does NOT look better on everybody, and is not necessarily more healthy. The real danger is that naturally non-slim women are endangering their health because they're told they could have a body like Naomi Campbell through diet and exercise (and very soon I expect to be much taller, with an insolent bottom, and rather black).

British *Slimmer* magazine headed an article called 'You can Change your Shape'. They defined only three body shapes – short and round (endomorph), lean and muscly (mesomorph) or tall and bony (ectomorph). The writers of the article ('famous for books and videos') say a short, round person can become leaner, and tall, bony people who do 'toning' exercises will 'become more shapely'. One person participating in the article who didn't like her hips had to do daily exercises, power walking three times a week and swimming three times a week. Of course she lost weight. But there was no proof given for her, or any others, that the basic body shape had changed.

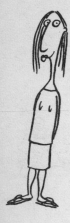

One of the strongest pushes from the shape-changing propagandists is the phrase 'body sculpting', heavy exercise of the kind that changed Madonna from a fleshy dancer into a hard-bodied one. If you concentrate on one or a few muscles, and work only on them, you will get a bigger, more defined muscle. That's why skaters develop bigger thighs and weightlifters bigger arms. Going the other way – making an area smaller by losing weight only from one specific area – is virtually undocumented.

'Body shape is not simply a gift from nature', claims the headline on a Clarins ad. 'Slim, firm contours and smooth skin result from a healthy lifestyle and daily care with specific, high-performance products.' These would presumably include the Contouring Body Cream and the Body Shaping Gel. The Contouring Cream does not contour, but tightens the skin while it is on, as egg white or glue does. The Body Shaping Gel does not shape your body, it is supposed to 'minimise the appearance of sponginess' by plumping out the skin. The Multi Mass Massage mitt, also advertised, is claimed to 'enhance firmness and tone' but it simply irritates the skin into temporary slight swelling which then looks smoother.

Remember: doctors disagree on exactly how many body types there are. But look around: there are as many as there are women. Or at least eight hundred and thirty seven.

The one thing almost all of the people who say you can change your shape have in common is that they are trying to sell you something.

Clothes sizes
Most clothes sizes have a variation of five centimetres. That means a size 12 in one label might fit you but a size 12 by another designer will feel too tight. At this point the sales assistant will say, 'It's European, dear', or 'It will shrink a bit when you wash it', or 'No, madam, this fabric never shrinks', or 'You'll grow into it', or 'You can lose half a stone', or 'Get out of the shop, you *monster*'. This is why elastic-waisted things are easy and why you should always try on something even if it says 'free size' or 'one size' or 'one size fits all'. (And by the way, can someone tell me why labels have 'small', 'medium' and 'large' for women and '1', '2', and '3' for men?)

International Clothes Sizes

British	8	10	12	14	16	18	20
Australian	8	10	12	14	16	18	20
French	36	38	40	42	44	46	48
Italian	38	40	42	44	46	48	50
German	34	36	38	40	42	44	46
American	6	8	10	12	14	16	18
Japanese	7	9	11	13			

In 1969 it was discovered that 86 per cent of women could be grouped into average sizes but there was also a need for variable fittings for fitted dresses and two-piece suits. Only 38 per cent would be fitted perfectly by the average sizes in each bust group; about one-quarter would need a slim hip fitting and one-quarter would need a fuller hip fitting.

Those extra fittings are no longer available. Instead, what we get in these mass-produced days are the restricted, plain average sizes without the variations that women need.

In Britain there is no set standard size coding scheme: it's a lottery. According to the British Fashion Council, retailers can set their own sizes and are free to alter them from season to season. If fashions are loose, sizes become smaller; if fashions are fitted, sizes get bigger. So whether you are a size 10 or a size 14 may depend on the whim of some fashion designer.

On the discovery that 47 per cent of British women are a size 16 or over, Helen Teague and Dawn French opened their shop *1647*, which sells clothes for this significant portion of the fashion-buying population. Nearly half of all women? That's quite a marketing potential! Hello? Is the fashion industry still awake?

A spokeswoman from *1647* said that in general we are getting bigger but manufacturers have added on a couple of inches to clothes sizes, so that we feel we are a size smaller. Some people think this is good marketing, as some women may be flattered into oblivion. 'You say I'm a size ten? Here – take all my money!'

The idea of size 12 being large rather than medium is a new one.

For years, size 12 women bought 'medium' clothes. Suddenly, without physically changing a millimetre, they were decreed 'large' by some manufacturers and labellers.

In her book *Being Fat is not a Sin*, English writer Shelley Bovey demonstrates how clothes sizes can be manipulated to make women feel flattered or estranged. The English size 14 used to be a medium, now it's a large. She says that in 1985 the Big Is Beautiful movement reported that 50 per cent of British women were a size 16 and over (large). Now that message has subtly changed to 60 per cent being size 14 and over. More than half of the female population were suddenly made 'large' by the stroke of a pen.

Bovey points out that in 1960 Marilyn Monroe 'epitomised all that was enviable to women and desirable to men. The little black dress she wore in *Some Like It Hot* was recently displayed in an exhibition of costumes. It was an outsize dress, a size 16.'

The clothes you see on models, even really tall ones, are usually size 10 or eight. One model agent says of designers, 'They only produce size 10 samples and a slim silhouette makes a wonderful clotheshorse'. Well tie her up, give her a handful of oats and see whether she whinnies.

Where to see normal

You will see only one type of normal in the magazines and on television and in films. That's the estimated 5 per cent of us, the model-shaped thin girls, with very long legs and wide shoulders. In years gone by we had actors ranging from Sophia Loren's shape to Mae West and back to feisty Katharine Hepburn and Rosalind Russell

Puberty was not kind. I grew taller, bigger and spottier than everybody in sixth class. I tried practically every weight-loss method invented. Sometimes I would lie in bed at night stupidly wishing some alien life form would kidnap me, free me of my fat (preferred alien method was by rolling down the fat off my body, like you would roll down stockings) and then return the slimmer, beautiful new me back to earth. Of course this never happened.

Susan, 24

Customer: So you haven't got anything in a size 14?
Assistant: They might have sent something by mistake. There's these...
Customer: They look a bit small to me.
Assistant: It's up to you, Porky.

Comedian, Victoria Wood

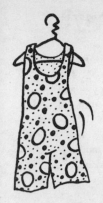

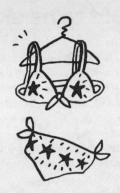

(check out the classics section at your video shop). British actors tend to have more diverse shapes but we see mostly the American ideal on our screens, which is the thinnest with the most make-up and the most fussed-over hair. It is also the most fiddled-with image, the most removed from reality, from the fake world.

We have to start looking at the real world again as well as watching the TV and reading the magazines. If we have our head stuck in that stuff all the time our idea of what is normal gets completely out of whack because we are only seeing the Five Per Cent. Go see women in the shopping mall. Oh my God! Where did all these real people come from? See how differently shaped they are?

See how the mothers and the women who have been through menopause look different? And if you really want to see life as it is, go and swim at a local pool or the beach or do an exercise class at a local gym, and have a look around you in the change room. Here we are. The 95 per cent. The 100 per cent. All different. Real gorgeous.

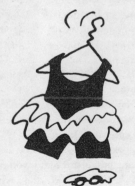

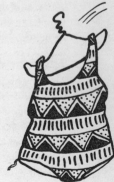

Why are we told to be skinny?

The freedom theory Thinness became a symbol of reproductive freedom, independence and youthful fun in the 1920s. The thinness ideal was born of women competing with men for jobs and opportunities: a denial of being seen as only fit for reproduction and decoration.

The health theory 'Thinner' always means 'healthier' and 'larger' automatically means 'less healthy'. Tell that to the tooth fairy.

The backlash theory

As women gain more political and economic power, the pressures on them to diet and be judged only by what they look like are intensified. This is part of the backlash against feminism. This theory is supported by Susan Faludi in her book *Backlash* and by Naomi Wolf in her book *The Beauty Myth*.

The fear of fat theory

There is prejudice against fat people. 'Excess body fat is probably the most stigmatised physical feature except skin colour,

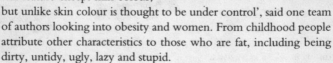

Many people assume I am anorexic because I am thin. In fact I probably eat more than other girls my age because everyone is always trying to fatten me up. I eat properly and am very active, and I find it insulting to be labelled anorexic. I have never even considered dieting. And in an effort to bolster up large girls' self-esteem, we thin girls are described as scrawny, waif-like, childlike and figureless. I may be petite, but I am every inch Woman!

Peta, 20

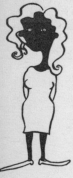

but unlike skin colour is thought to be under control', said one team of authors looking into obesity and women. From childhood people attribute other characteristics to those who are fat, including being dirty, untidy, ugly, lazy and stupid.

The media theory The media cover the different variations of the communications industry, including press, film and television. These media have set up an impossible, glamorous ideal and censor most other images of real women by excluding them. For example,

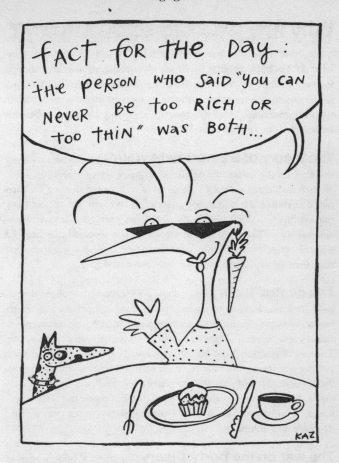

a male reporter can be bald and fat as long as his work is satisfactory, but a woman newsreader on a commercial channel cannot even change her hair colour without permission. The newsreader is telling us that half of Zaire just got arrested and we wonder why she's wearing that weird blouse.

The eternal youth theory Thinness in girls reaches a peak at about the age of 12, just before the body changes of puberty. Some people think that women who want to remain very thin also do not really want to grow up. Many of the models used to display heavy make-up and low-cut gowns are in fact 12- and 13-year-olds who have not yet been through the body change ingeniously disguised as women. Older women are fearful of age, character lines, hair that gets darker and then turns grey; younger women are afraid of the changes that puberty brings, afraid to grow up, knowing that a pre-pubescent body is the one most glorified.

The theory of learned behaviour

Monkey see, monkey do. Part of the initiation of growing up, part of watching adult women and learning how to be an adult, is learning that we are supposed to dislike our bodies, or at least bits of them. Or at least have one bit that you don't like (pick a part, any part). A *Glamour* magazine survey of 33,000 of its American readers revealed that only 13 per cent of respondents thought that their mothers were satisfied with their bodies. (Fathers were not considered.)

The control theory

Fat people are most often wrongly seen to have 'let themselves go'. In a world where they do not have very much power, some people take pride in conquering their body's natural needs and being in 'control'. Seeming to be in control is seen to be a virtue. This is why people talk of punishing themselves with exercise or with guilt for performing a natural function such as being hungry and eating. 'I can't control my life but I can control my eating', is a common feeling of someone with an eating disorder. (Unfortunately this really translates to, 'I can't control my life but I sure as hell can control getting more miserable and unhealthy'.)

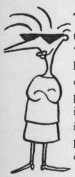

The war on the body theory

The natural body is seen as the enemy. The *Utne Reader* magazine in America put it this way, 'We have declared war on our bodies...our over-worked, high-speed lifestyles have severed any relationship between our bodies and the cycles of nature, including the body's own natural rhythms'. This is part of the reason plastic surgeons think they can get away with saying small breasts are 'deformed'. Technology is always good and any invention should be tried out but the natural body is bad, defective, primitive, must be made to submit to drugs, obsessive dieting, being cut open and having foreign bodies inserted.

The femininity theory

Old-fashioned notions of 'fem-ininity' suggested that a woman should not eat well, but 'like a bird', be fragile, quiet (squeaky, even), modest, powerless, sup-portive and retiring – in short 'ladylike'. She should make and serve food for others but hold back on eating herself. This lack of appetite is often seen to apply to other wants such as ambition, self-fulfilment, personal pursuits.

> I think most girls and ladies think they are the wrong shape and are fat because these days it's supposedly in to be very thin. It's put across in magazines, TV, all media to look like the small per cent of people who model. I think to fix this problem magazines, TV etc. should have more 'normal'-sized models modelling.
>
> Naomi, 12

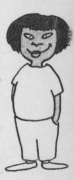

The brainwash theory
Fashion arbiters, magazine editors and beauty and fashion writers are all participating in the relentless brainwashing that thin is good. The designers only provide samples in size ten. Feeling guilty about this, and doing what they can to redress the balance, the magazines try to run positive stories about self-esteem and body image, and end up with a confusing collage of opposing messages.

The capitalism theory
The trend to more and more thin-ness as an ideal has coincided with the rise of women as an econom-ically powerful group. There are more young, single women delaying marriage and childbirth or rejecting both options altogether, with 'disposable income' to spend on themselves. There is extra money to be made from such women, as well as from women who can be made to feel that they are 'losing their looks' through drudgery and age. The easiest way to sell people something is to convince them they need it: so the campaigns denigrate the most common shape of women as unsightly or unwanted. Not much money can be made by telling women there isn't anything wrong with them and they don't need to buy anything to fix it. The 'You're too fat' message is mar-keting, not fact.

The duty theory
It is a duty for women to 'make the best of themselves', to show men that they want their approval. Submitting to

this is supposed to be part of a woman's lot. This theory is encouraged by those who sell cosmetics and want you to pay £50 to be wrapped in some plankton and clingfilm as a useless cellulite 'treatment'.

Probably a mix of many or all of these theories contribute to the imposed thin ideal. (Also it may have something to do with aliens and strange circles in wheat paddocks. This would be part of the Gullible Loony Theory.)

How do you judge your size and shape?

American cartoonist Nicole Hollander says: 'My weight is perfect for my height, which varies.'

According to one respected eating disorders doctor, in Sydney, Australia, 'Any weight you feel comfortable with is the right weight. Things like the pinch test are a load of garbage.'

Body Mass Index The Body Mass Index is one way of assessing weight but is not a suitable test for anyone less than 18 years old.

The way you find your BMI is to get your calculator, or your brain if you're a maths whiz, find your weight in kilograms and your height in metres squared (sorry girls, it only works in metric!). Now divide your *weight* by your *height squared*. For example, if you weigh 52 kilos and your height is 1.58 metres, squared it's 2.4964. You divide 2.4964 into 52 and get 20.829. That answer 20.8 is your Body Mass Index.

Underweight is defined as a BMI of less than 20, acceptable as 20 to 25, overweight as 26 to 30 and obese, as more than 30. According to the Bureau, women were less likely than men to be overweight and more likely to be underweight.

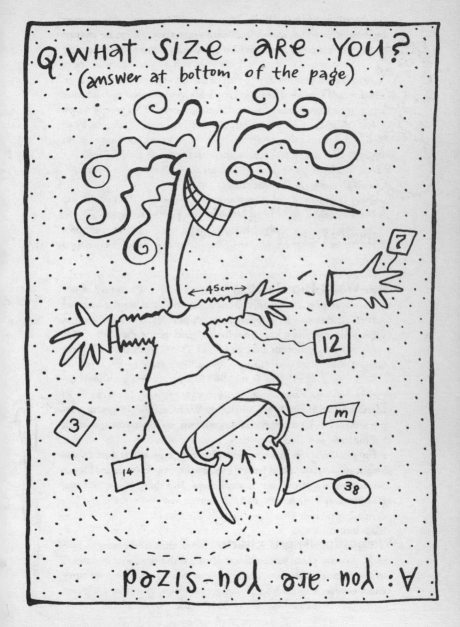

Most young women (18 to 24 years) who were not at an acceptable weight were underweight. Nearly one-third of young women were underweight and only 8.1 per cent were overweight, and only 2.8 per cent were obese. Yet people in this age group were more likely to diet than others.

In *Eating Disorders: The Facts* Derek Llewellyn-Jones and Suzanne Abraham add two extra categories: gross obesity (BMI over 40) and emaciated (BMI under 15), putting the normal weight range as 19 to 25. But the main thing to remember is not to get too hung up on numbers. And if you're a teenager, resist the temptation of applying the BMI test to yourself – it's irrelevant unless you've definitely stopped growing (in any direction!)

Other doctors say that overweight is defined as a BMI in the top 15 per cent of the population, no matter what the score is.

The big problem with the Body Mass Index is that it ignores where the fat is on the body, the fact that muscle weighs more than fat, and genes.

The Waist-Hip Ratio A better measure of whether your shape is healthy is the amount of flesh around your waist compared to your hips. If you have been through puberty and your waist is bigger than your hips, you may be in need of some exercise. (Or you may be five months pregnant, I can't tell from here.) If your waist is smaller than your hips you most likely have no problems.

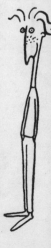

To get your Waist–Hip Ratio (WHR) you divide your *waist circumference* by the *hip circumference*. For example, if your waist is 30 inches and your hips are 39 inches your WHR is 0.77. In young children a WHR of 1.1 is common, going down to 0.8 for young women after puberty.

The Hip–Waist Ratio is used to determine people at greater risk of heart disease later in life: this is where the beer belly (waist bigger than hips) really shows up as dangerous. In other words, hips are good for you, 'beer bellies' bad.

Weight-for-height charts Ignore most of the weight-for-height charts you see on the back of packets of stockings and tights or in racks at the chemist. Some of them have been reprinted from tables put together decades ago and are no longer considered relevant or accurate. The more specific a chart is, the less useful it is.

The weight-for-height charts do not take into account that muscle weighs more than fat, that everyone weighs more as they get older, once they have stopped growing, water retention due to hormonal cycles, or that the definitions of acceptable weight can change. One researcher at the US National Institute on Aging says the charts are relevant only for people in their early forties.

At 30, I am 15 stone, most of which is muscle, but certainly not all. I come from large-boned European ancestors and consider myself to be fairly strong and healthy-looking. Men don't seem to have been put off by my non-stereotype body – I've had a fair few long-term relationships, sexual flings and offers. I must say the one thing about not being a '10' is that the guys you get with (the serious ones) are attracted by you as a person right from the start, not superficial attraction fuelled by magazine hype.

Anne

Weight-for-height charts should include a *range* of healthy weights, for example from six and a half to eight and a half stone, not an individual number such as seven and a half stone. This allows for the wide diversity of human beings who are all different and don't always fit neatly onto charts and into statistics. Not to mention their trousers.

Body fat percentage

Women need about 17 per cent of their body weight as fat in order to menstruate and about 22 per cent fat in order to have regular menstrual cycles. Below 20 per cent is the average at which women stop having periods.

Doctors involved in athletics accept 14 to 20 per cent body fat on women. *The Beauty Myth* by Naomi Wolf says that from birth girls have 10 to 15 per cent more fat than boys. The average healthy 20-year-old female has 28.7 per cent body fat. By middle age, women cross-culturally have about 38 per cent body fat.

Wondering why those shop dummies have such thin hips? They haven't started menstruating (what a thought). No, really, a study of shop mannequins has shown they have been getting thinner since the 1950s, and the modern ones, if they were real women, would not have enough body fat on them to menstruate.

The right size and shape for you

If you eat healthy food and have a few indulgences every now and again and if you also exercise three times a week for more than half an hour, you are at the size and shape you should be. This formula is agreed by doctors, nutritionists, and body-image consultants. If anybody tells you any different, they're either misled or trying to sell you something. You may shout at them.

Further reading

Angela Phillips and Jill Rakusen, *The New Our Bodies Ourselves* (2nd edition, Penguin Books, 1989). A fantastic reference, a huge soft-cover book all about the natural female body, how it works, what it looks like, common ailments and what to do about them.

Edward Shorter, *A History of Women's Bodies* (Penguin Books, 1984)

Naomi Wolf, *The Beauty Myth* (Vintage, 1991)

Susan Faludi, *Backlash—The Undeclared War against Women* (Vintage, 1993)

Shelley Bovey, *Forbidden Body: Why Being Fat is not a Sin* (Pandora, 1994)

chapter *two*

Weight for me

Food

Food as a sin 'Oh, I mustn't', 'Oh, I really shouldn't', 'It will go straight to my hips'. I guess we're just not encouraged to say, 'Oh, no, I couldn't possibly. It would go straight to the production of skin cells, my central nervous system, and my toenail growth'. (Normal body functioning accounts for 70 per cent of daily energy expenditure.)

Slimmer magazine has a 'Shapescope' astrology column which in one month tells Aquarians that they have a body like an intricate machine and are told not to neglect their health (as if) and Scorpios they are going to meet someone new so they'd better lose weight. Pisces must say 'no' to temptation in October. In fact there is an awful lot about temptation: Librans should only have romance as a temptation if they lose weight; Aries need willpower; Geminis need determination *and* willpower (they're not eating for two, after all) and Leos shouldn't be giving in to tasty titbits. Virgos, too must not give in to temptation.

Australia's *Cleo* magazine's survey 'Love, Sex and the Dieting Woman' found that 67 per cent of women feel guilty every day about eating.

According to diet lore, 'indulging' or 'giving in to temptation' is

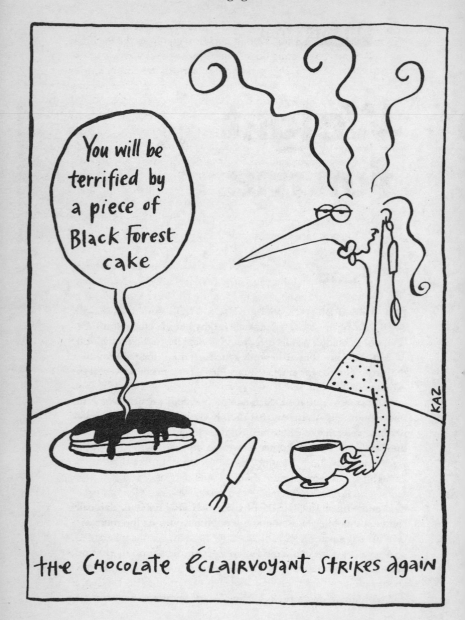

a 'sin'. (Strangling a few people is a sin. Invading East Timor is a sin. 'Ethnic cleansing' is a sin. Testing nuclear weapons in the Pacific is a sin. I'm sorry, but eating doesn't quite make the grade.)

Australian *Who Weekly* magazine, which has run many stories about eating disorders, kicked off 1994 with its front cover screamer 'Diet Winners and Sinners of the Year: here's the scoop on who got fat, who got fit and how they did it'.

Comedian Jennifer Saunders says, 'I'm completely neurotic about [weight]. I've always been overweight. Actually I haven't always been overweight. I started as soon as I became this moody sort of schoolgirl…I put on weight and then dieted at school. Cup of soup for lunch and then you'd go across to the shop and buy six Mars Bars. No-one's teaching you anything: you should just eat normally. Just be sane about it. Not like these neurotic people who go, "Well, that's a bit naughty isn't it, what you're eating?" Naughty! I'm eating! It's food. I'm EATING IT…I KNOW I'M BEING NAUGHTY. EATING FOOD IS WRONG ALTOGETHER'.

> If I'm out to dinner and everyone orders a dessert, I order one too. What I've learned to do is just take two bites and push the plate away. After all, you don't have to eat everything on your plate. Normally my husband finishes it off!
>
> Cindy Crawford, American model

Seven thousand respondents to a *Mirabella* magazine survey in the US revealed that those who were extremely overweight ate the most lollies but at 47 per cent, the dangerously *underweight* ate more cakes and cookies than anyone else. The most craved foods were chocolate and ice-cream. Chocolate is seen as the biggest sin and so consequently it is the biggest craving.

The gender gap: show us your portion
Traditionally food is served in its best and largest proportions to the men: as a reward for status, as fuel for hunting. Biscuits, like handkerchiefs, come in 'man size'. Little children in countries where there is not enough food will have more chance of survival if they are boys: they are given more food. Having a smaller portion used to be seen as ladylike, dainty, mysterious. Fanatical Christian girls were praised in

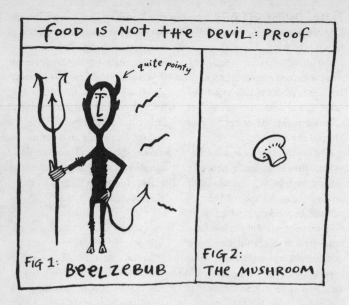

FIG 1: BEELZEBUB — food is not the devil: proof — quite pointy

FIG 2: THE MUSHROOM

years gone by for refusing to eat, fainting and having hallucinations (visions from the Lord). Their wasted bodies were seen as proof that they could live on faith alone. To be thin and deprived was to be 'good'.

Food as a reward Eating is often associated with reward in our society – an ice-cream for being good, lollies after eating our 'greens', a celebratory meal, a birthday cake. Food gets mixed up with love or with comfort and security for some people. Cooking is often an act of love and nourishment from a parent or lover and it becomes symbolic of being cared for and protected.

The smell or appearance of food 'induces an anticipatory increase in insulin (blood sugar) – and in appetite', say Peter Dally and Joan Gomez, authors of *Understanding Anorexia and Obesity*. 'The pleasurable feelings associated with the beginning of a meal are due to endorphins, self-made opiates which give a sense of well-being. For most people the endorphin concentration falls away quickly as the meal progresses.'

Food pornography The glossy, full-colour pictures of chocolate cakes and fruit custard flans in magazines that also carry diets is a forbidden realm but an irresistible one. One ice-cream is described in sexual advertising as 'wicked'. Another is 'to die for'. Denial of food is strongly linked to an obsession with it. Some anorexics and bulimics throw elaborate dinner parties, worship food, become 'foodies'. They cannot eat it or absorb it but they must be near it. It's a kind of masochistic torture.

> I read an article by a leading women's nutritionist which said that any guilt feelings about eating certain types of foods could be described as an eating disorder. Well, that's me to a T! A bundle of guilt feelings. I love chocolate more than any other food (except maybe tortellini) and I have convinced myself that this is the source of all my problems. I have tried everything to cut down on the choccy habit – the latest is to add up the money I've saved from resisting temptation and buy something as a reward. This seems to make it even harder to resist and I get into a terrible tizz about it all and if I break down and eat some chocolate I feel so bad about myself.
>
> Margaret

Food obsession Most diet books encourage the food obsession. Margaret O'Sullivan's *The Heavenly Body Diet Book* suggests that women keep a 'food diary'.

'It's absolutely essential,' she said while promoting her book. 'It takes me no more than three minutes and I do it in bed at night or during the commercial breaks when I'm watching television.' She, too, talks of 'keeping your weight under control' by counting calories weekly rather than daily. This she sees as an incredible freedom!

'If you indulge every now and again you simply take extra care on the other days.' This hardly revolutionary idea, along with its boring calorie-counting obsession, was promoted on almost a full page of a national Sunday paper.

Maybe it started with that weirdo Bible story. I mean, a

> I eat normally for a few months until I find the enthusiasm or mental strength to starve myself again. I find it really difficult as I love my food too much and I can't bear to miss out on it for too long.
>
> Louise, 19

woman eats an apple – one little apple! And the next thing
you know everyone's chucked
out of the garden of Eden and
all the evils of the earth, including lawyers and public transport
ticket inspectors, famine and
pestilence, are visited upon the
earth by a vengeful and furious
all-powerful God. No wonder
women feel guilty about eating.
Thankfully Eve wasn't offered
a piece of black forest cake by
that old snakie thing or we'd all be pulverised into atoms.

> I began losing weight. I was eight and a
> half stone in Year 3 and by the time Year 5
> began I was just over six stone and every-
> one told me how good I looked. I lost
> interest in food. My eating habits are still
> appalling. Today I've had a donut,
> Maltesers, pizza, Coke and three oranges.
> I really worry about my kids adopting my
> eating habits.
>
> Kim, 24

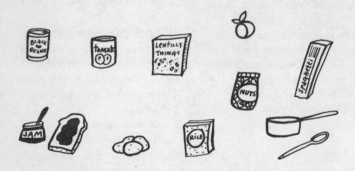

Nutrition

Healthy eating The top-selling item at British supermarkets is
Coca Cola. I hope you were not expecting it to be unprocessed bran,
kelp byproducts or agar agar. No, the British are more your sort of
Coco Pops nutritionists.

So, if we assume that we should not be drinking eight litres of
Coke and having a lardburger every couple of hours, how *should* we
be eating?

An Eating Behaviours project suggests some ideas for healthier eating:

- Give yourself permission to eat.
- 'Legalise' all foods without feeling guilt.
- Avoid counting calories.
- Use hunger as the cue for eating, not the time of day or habit.
- Eat small meals about every three to five hours.
- Trust your food choices – eat anything you want, forbid nothing.
- Sit down while eating.
- Don't hide away and eat alone – create a pleasant environment and table to eat at.
- Focus your senses on food, its colour, smell, texture, and taste. (They also mention sounds but if your food is singing, put it away.)
- Notice how your body reacts to certain foods.

There are not many rules for healthy eating, but here they are:

- Don't diet: ever.
- Eat what your body wants you to.
- Vary your food so you don't get bored.
- Don't stick popcorn up your nose.
- Don't trust food advertising.
- Know where your food comes from.
- Don't use added salt.
- Eat fresh food whenever possible.
- Eat as much organically produced food as you can afford.
- If you get into a food fight, make sure you have the custard.

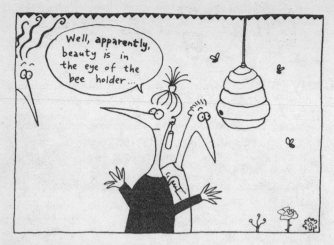

Well, apparently, beauty is in the eye of the bee holder...

The food groups Forget the old five food groups you learned years ago – they have been modified. Modified, hell, nutrition's a completely different beastie.

Don't take any notice of the magazine that said, 'Peruse your plate and leave something on it. There's no reason to eat all the food you're served just because it's there. Your main course arrives with chicken, roast pumpkin and green beans. Eat two of the three choices and leave the third one after a little taste.' Noooooooooooo! Eat some of all three!

Our body needs regular hits of the following things: water; vitamins A, C, D, E, K and B complex; calcium, iron, folic acid; magnesium, iron; zinc; phosphorus; potassium; sodium (no need to add it, it's in most foods already); sulphur; iodine; complex carbohydrates; protein; essential fatty acids; and fibre. The key is in eating a *variety* of foods to get all the goodies.

> How could anorexia be so bad? Once I lose the weight I want, I'll keep going so if I pig out I don't gain fat, I gain weight. Then I'll be able to stop – I can't go without food for long, think of all the white chocolate and glazed donuts!
>
> Summer

Generally, we tend to have too much fat, alcohol, sugar, salt, and animal protein and not enough green, leafy things, vegetables, fruit, bread and grains.

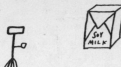

Daily needs Meats and meat alternatives – including

fish, the odd egg, nuts, seeds – once a day (go easy on the salami!), twice for a woman who is pregnant, for extra iron, zinc and protein.

Milk and dairy products – including cheese and yoghurt – 2 portions (this could be a glass of milk and a small tub of yoghurt). Pregnant women need 3 portions for extra protein and calcium.

Veggies – you know, the stuff at the greengrocer's. Go wild and eat lots but have at least 4 portions of different veggies a day. Lentils and legumes are included here.

Fruit – 'An apple a day…' Fresh is best – 3 different types a day.

Breads and cereals – important for fibre. Include rice and pasta. Go for it with 5 and preferably more portions a day. (Not so difficult when a portion is a slice of bread or half a cup of cereal.) Pregnant and active women may need 7 to 8 portions a day. Very active adults and growing teenagers can need up to 9 to 12 portions a day (preferably wholemeal).

And remember, a cakie a day keeps the madness away.

This is a loose guide only: you don't want to be weighing bits of food and counting up slices and generally getting obsessed with it. Food is not mathematics. Life is too short to weigh lentils.

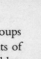

I like this idea the best: Many nutritionists just divide the food groups into three sections: eat less fat, oil and sugar; moderate amounts of meat fish, poultry, eggs and dairy foods; and lots of fruit, vegetables, legumes, bread and cereals. How simple is that?

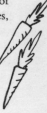

You'll find that this is probably what your body is asking for once it settles down anyway. You'll be lying there and your body will say, 'I'd like some spinach and something kind of crunchy, maybe in a more lurid shade of orange.' 'A carrot?' you'll inquire. 'That's it,' the body will say. 'I'll have a couple of those carroty things and something red and round and deliciously squishy that explodes in your mouth.' 'I believe that's what they refer to in intellectual circles as a cherry tomato,' you'll reply. 'And I want a cheese sandwich and a Polo. Later I may toy with leeks.'

If somebody hassles you about eating too much, or eating between meals, strike them repeatedly with this book.

Osteoporosis

This is a deficiency disease. The bones lose minerals, particularly calcium, and become brittle and weak, often causing stooping and breaking bones in old age. The decline in bone strength tends to speed up after menopause. Technically, the term refers to people who have lost 50 to 75 per cent of their original bone material. Although generally we are told, especially by dairy organisations, that dairy food calcium intake is the key to protecting ourselves, excessive animal protein consumption, including milk consumption, has been linked to osteoporosis.

The average measurable bone loss in a woman meat-eater at 65 years old in America is 35 per cent. The average rate for her vegetarian sister at the same age: 7 per cent. It seems that the more animal protein we eat (including that from fish), the more calcium our bodies lose.

Unchallenged research shows that even very high calcium intakes are cancelled out by high animal protein consumption. Bantu women have a dangerously low calcium intake by our standards, but they eat virtually no animal protein. Their

> I used food to make me feel better when I was in a state of discomfort. I am now in my healthy weight range and I have worked hard to break the relationship with food and comfort. Now food is for nutrition.
>
> Millie, 24

osteoporosis rate is very low. This doesn't mean we should stop taking in calcium: we still need it. But it would seem that rather than simply eating more dairy products, we should be eating less protein supplied by meat.

Physical activity from a young age is also linked to low rates of osteoporosis, so get dancing.

Further information

To know about which foods have which goodies, a visit to a community dietitian or a good book on different foods might be useful. There are also a number of useful leaflets and pamphlets produced by large retailers and food companies – don't forget to send a stamped, addressed envelope.

British Nutrition Foundation
High Holborn House
52-54 High Holborn
London WC1V 6RQ

Phone (0171) 404 6504

Further reading

Peter Cox, *The Realeat Encyclopedia of Vegetarian Living* (Bloomsbury, 1994)

Susan Kano, *Never Diet Again* (Thorsons, 1994)

Dieting

On a diet? The world is full of girls and women eating only fruit until midday, following diets that claim to shed weight from the hips, thighs and left earlobe only, chatting with a fake smile to cover the growling of their stomachs. They are looking wistfully at packets of chocolate biscuits, eating crispbread that tastes like boiled cardboard, counting up kilojoules, feeling desperate and miserable, and wondering why they're insanely hungry. They are on a diet and it won't work.

> I want to be 47 kilos.
> I would be happy at 47 kilos.
>
> Marla, 20

Up to 66 per cent of British women diet sporadically and 15 per cent are on permanent diets, according to *Options* magazine. Ninety-five per cent of dieters regain their lost weight. A study in Bristol found 1 in 55 women between the ages of 15 and 25 had an eating disorder. Many are depriving themselves of almost all the 2000 kilo-calories of energy needed each day to maintain the body functions of a healthy woman. Even those depriving themselves of 'eating between meals' are missing out on the essential supply of the 2000 kilocalories spread across their waking hours.

Why diets make you gain weight I don't mean that diets don't work because you never lose weight but that the weight is almost always regained. *Not* because you don't have enough willpower but because the body and the mind have special powers to deal with the starvation you are putting yourself through. When you diet, you do lose some weight – not fat, but water and muscle. This dehydration makes you weigh less and look thinner for a little while. Then the body insists you have to eat something. Your mind is obsessed with food, it screams out for you to feed yourself. Meanwhile the body reacts by saving fat and storing more every time you eat.

Every time you lose weight, your body goes into coping mode for

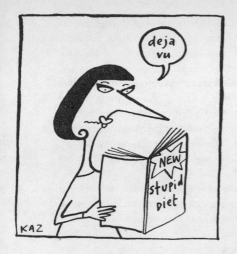

starvation. The metabolism slows down so you burn off less fat. The body re-educates itself to work on less food. Valuable muscle tissue, not fat, is eaten away. Food cravings begin, leading to overeating, binge-eating, or eating of low-use high-sugar foods such as snack food and chocolate bars. The body stores away more fat, having been programmed now to expect starvation or famine again.

Get this: if you diet, you are actually training your body to become fatter as a protection against further dieting. Your body is an utter smarty-pants.

'The final result is that some women who started off at a good weight-for-height ratio, over a period of ten or 20 years have steadily increased their weight, size and fat percentage to a point of no return. Obesity then, can be caused by constant dieting and the following weight gain,' says community nurse Penelope Goward.

Willpower schmillpower. There is nothing wrong with *you* – there's a lot wrong with dieting. To recover we must listen to our bodies, not work against them. Except in the case of an illness or a disorder, your body knows what it is doing. It has been genetically programmed to do it for thousands of years and no short-term starvation magazine diet can get the better of it.

So what is the secret? The only way is to work *with* the body, by

> Diet pills: I tried the ones you buy at the chemist at age 15. I lost the few pounds I wanted to, but looking back I really didn't need to lose any weight. I think people need to accept their shape and as this happens they will begin to accept other people's shapes. It would be a boring old world if everyone had the body of an iron man or supermodel.
>
> Teri, 22

feeding it healthy food and a few indulgences and exercising as regularly as possible. People who are not obsessed with food, not dieting, not feeling hungry and deprived, accept themselves as they are and live happier lives.

The generally accepted percentage of dieters who regain the weight they have lost is about 95 per cent. (This figure is from a study called 'Obesity' by the Royal College of Physicians.) Other figures of 90 per cent and 98 per cent have been mentioned but I suspect they may be estimates. The dieting industry certainly doesn't want to publicise the extraordinarily high rate of failure of their programs and potions.

Those who regain the weight they lose do so within two years of their weight-loss programs according to a study by the University of Texas. The study found that when people were taught to eat as they wished, they gained self-confidence and better health (but more of that later).

The body *needs* the extra padding on thighs, hips and bottoms (where women want to lose it) and will protect itself against starvation. Your body is looking after you, even while you are abusing it. Imagine what it could be like if you worked together.

Dieting makes you sick 'Dieting, losing weight and putting it back on again is far worse than maintaining a heavy weight,' says Dr Jane Ogden, author of *Fat Chance!* The stress put on the body by the starvation and sudden eating, and the resultant dramatic changes is very unhealthy, threatening your immune system and the general workings of your body and its organs. It will also cause stretch marks. The healthy, gradual weight loss that happens on a healthy, abundant diet along with exercise should be no more than two pounds a week.

Dieting makes you depressed Because dieting doesn't work, people blame a lack of willpower. Dieters blame themselves when they had only a 5 per cent chance of success in the first place: less if they had dieted before. By its very nature, dieting makes people unsatisfied, wanting, yearning, unfulfilled. Hunger is depressing.

> I weigh four and a half stone more than I'd like. I have been fat since I was four years old. I have always been a healthy eater – I eat all the right things, not a lot. There was a succession of diets from age four: none worked. I tried calorie-counting diets, magazine diets, doctor diets, acupuncture, laser treatment, prescribed drugs, diet drinks, Gloria Marshall, Easyslim, Weight Watchers, Jenny Craig. Nothing has worked. So I am still fat.
>
> Melissa, 22

Not being able to enjoy food is depressing. Being terrified of a carrot is so extremely depressing I don't even want to think about it.

Dieting makes you obsessed with food

Penelope Goward explains: 'If you lower your calories (as in a diet) the psychical signal your body gets is "starvation" or "famine" and responds accordingly. No one can exist on a reduced food intake without exhibiting a "starvation" response. This over-interest is a normal part of feeling physically hungry every 3 to 5 hours – we instinctively want to feed ourselves. There is increased interest in food which over a period of prolonged dieting can become an induced food obsession – like food fantasies, food dreams, waiting for your next meal, talking about food, planning meals and generally finding food on your mind for most of the time.'

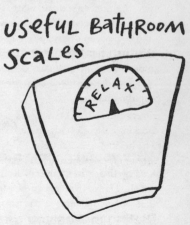

useful Bathroom scales

Dieting makes you unhealthy

Dr Dale Atrens pointed out in his book *Don't Diet* that the futile pursuit of dieting makes people believe that they cannot lose weight because they haven't the willpower. So they give up attempts to start regular exercise, think they might as well smoke and drink, and eat lots of sugary foods under the mistaken impression that their extra weight necessarily makes them unhealthy. In fact their weight may be perfectly natural and healthy for them.

Penelope Goward says that continued dieting makes your body exhibit signs and symptoms of poor nutrition such as extreme hunger, irritability, depression and anxiety, nervousness, fatigue, listlessness, poor sleep patterns, desire for sugar and poor concentration.

> I took diet pills. At night I would dream of food, and I stopped taking them and went up to size 16. Then I didn't think about weight gain and started to lose weight. I'm size 12–14 now and I'm quite happy with myself. In Europe now it's okay to be big: big women walk around in bikinis, and no one cares.
>
> Gillian, 19

One then finally has to give in to eating, the natural survival instinct.

Dieting makes you stupid A British study of dieting students showed that they performed much worse than a group of normal eaters when tested on reaction times, rapid information processing and memory. Doctors believe that part of the problem was the dieters were so obsessed with food and body image they could not concentrate effectively on other tasks. The lack of food was also a shock to the system, causing stress, which reduces concentration and ability to focus. Another explanation would be that diets induce lowered heart rates or starve the brain of glucose. The women who did the least well in the tests were the ones who had been dieting the longest.

Why young people must not diet Teenagers being hassled by their parents about their eating should show them this paragraph. *Dieting is dangerous for young people.* Not quite as dangerous as removing your brain and setting fire to it, but pretty close.

These are your growth spurt years. You need the growth, you need the brain power and you need the energy that good food gives you. You don't need the hassle of dieting. Overweight young people need good food and exercise. But are you really overweight? If you are eating good food and exercising for at least half an hour three

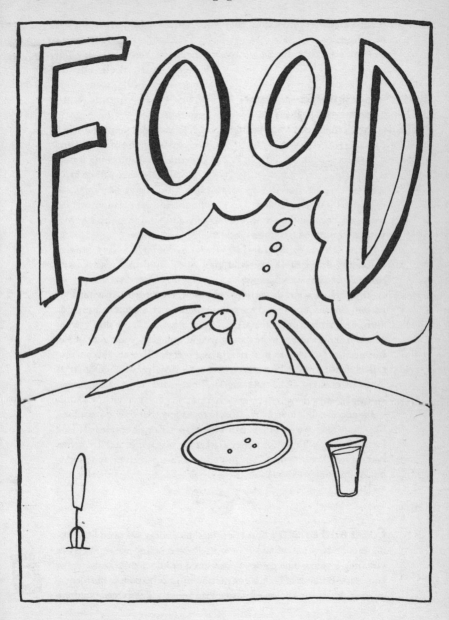

times a week (even walking) then your body will be at the right size and shape.

Here's another thing to show the naggers. *You should be eating between meals*. Well, hurrah! Some soya milk, some sunflower seeds, yoghurt, fruit, vegetables or a whole-grain cheese and salad sandwich when you get home from school and something mid-morning is fine. This will help stave off the craving for junk food, like chips and chocolate, very dangerous for teenagers because they're so easy to buy and so unhealthy for you, with all the added fats, sugar and salt.

> So what's the diet? Well you eat a hard-boiled egg before every meal and the hard-boiled egg actually eats some of that meal for you.
>
> Comedian Victoria Wood

Jenny O'Dea, dietitian and lecturer at Sydney University, studied the eating habits of 13-year-old girls. She found that regardless of size, 42 per cent were dieting.

'But dieting is not the answer,' she said. 'Dieting in growing adolescents impairs growth and restricts nutrients such a protein, iron, calcium and zinc, which teenagers need a lot of. You don't want children and teenagers to be losing weight unless they are very obese. It is normal for them to gain height and weight. Parents also need to realise that it's normal for girls to put on a large percentage of fat. A lot of parents say, "She's getting fat," but really she's just getting a womanly shape.'

Parents can also help by reassuring teenagers that they do not look like enormous space-porkers from the Planet Zorg but normal-sized human beings who are the target market for magazines and TV shows with pretend young people in pretend make-up with pretend lighting and pretend personalities.

Food and energy Food provides the energy we need for making our body function and renew itself even while we're asleep or watching a video. The energy is measured in kilocalories (calories) or kilojoules. Because of their faster metabolism, some people burn energy (or calories, or kilojoules) faster than others. Teenagers, children,

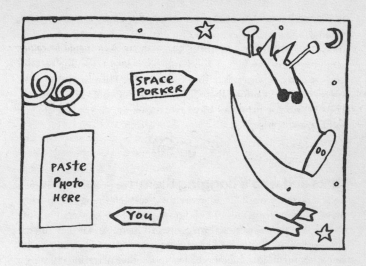

pregnant women and naturally larger people generally need more energy.

Calories and kilojoules are calculated from the composition of different foods. For example, a gram of fat gives 37 kilojoules (9 kcal), a gram of alcohol 29 kilojoules (7 kcal) and a gram of carbohydrate provides 16 kilojoules (4 kcal).

According to the British Nutrition Foundation, successful weight loss requires a moderate reduction in energy intake – eating 500 kilocalories less than your body needs will result in weight loss of about 1lb (1/2 kg) per week. Some short-term diets such as fasts and fruit or liquid diets are below starvation levels of kilojoule intake.

It makes you feel guilty about everything you eat. Seems skinny people just are better than you because they can stay on a diet. Girlfriends have the biggest influence, they are who you compare yourselves to, if they can lose weight and stay thin and you can't you feel lower than them. What I would give to look like a magazine model. Bodywise, your face is your own individuality coming out but everyone's got the same body or can have. I would want Cindy Crawford's body.

Kylie

The trouble with counting calories or kilojoules is that it ignores vitamins and minerals and makes no distinction between whether or not you've had any greens in the last calendar year. It encourages an obsession with tiny bits of food and discourages listening to your body to find out what it is telling you it needs. There are many other considerations in eating apart from simple kilojoule consumption. How big are you naturally? How much exercise do you do? Do you feel like an icy pole?

Diets and who's flogging them
The people who sell diets *know* they don't work. That's why they keep churning out so many 'new' ones in magazines. They know people are desperate to lose weight, and they have to sell magazines to them. And if they run the same healthy nutrition and exercise recommendation in every magazine, they might lose gullible readers to another magazine claiming a 'revolution' or a 'breakthrough'. They know that young readers are influenced and want to look like models. Even though the magazines know that is an impossible dream, they will run 'supermodel diets'.

Every diet that isn't a plan for general nutrition is a fad diet. Dietitian Jo Rogers, who worked for 40 years at the Royal Prince Alfred Hospital, on her retirement let fly at fad diets, naming the '*Women's Weekly* Wonder Diet' promoted by former model and spokeswoman Maggie Tabberer as promoting 'nutritional quackery'.

Ms Tabberer said the diet was only meant to be short-term but Jo Rogers was having none of it. 'Maggie Tabberer's Wonder Diet was close to a starvation diet and it isn't going to teach people anything, because everyone knows if they starve they'll lose weight. Maggie claims it's to give you a 'kick start' but that's not helpful because it just involves loss of fluid. As soon as you resume normal eating you regain the weight and then people become disappointed in themselves,' she told *Who Weekly* magazine.

'In a successful weight-loss program weight loss will be slow. We need to overcome our obsession with weight and make the best of what we are. The plan should be supported by 30 minutes of exercise three times weekly.'

Who Weekly asked, 'If I needed to shed five kilograms fast to fit

> I have tried water diets, no breakfast diets, no lunch diets, no dinner diets, no food diets. But none work! Because I don't have the willpower. There's a lot of food I don't like so I can't take diets out of the magazines.
>
> Sybilla, 17

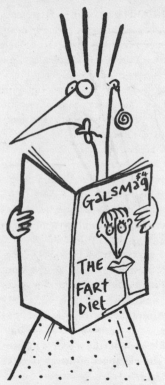

into a slinky cocktail dress, what would you suggest?' That's easy. 'Buy another dress,' replied Jo Rogers.

A doctors' magazine asked a panel of four nutritionists to evaluate seven diets in women's magazines published in 1993. Only one was approved, the only diet to take account of recommended daily vitamins and minerals and to encourage a healthy long-term eating plan.

Four of the diets recommended in the women's magazines had less than half the required energy for a woman aged 20 to 30, and were low in important vitamins and minerals, especially iron and zinc.

Professor of dietetics and nutrition, David Roberts said the first day of Maggie's Wonder Diet would be more like the diarrhoea diet on day one, followed by farting for day two, diarrhoea *and* farting on day three and constipation on the rice-only day four. Charming. The low-carbohydrate diets would result in the body losing water, muscle tissue and 'pretty well' no fat, according to nutritionist Rosemary Stanton.

Australian Doctor concluded, 'The panellists agreed that women's magazines would continue to publish diets that were anti-social, unpalatable, inflexible, nutritionally unbalanced and that did not consider cost, food availability or the person's likes and dislikes.' Basically, the short-term diets in magazines are crap.

Perhaps the dumbest diets are the single-food diets, like the Maggie Tabberer one, or the Israeli Army diet (only apples one day, only cheese another), the Beverly Hills Diet, the Grapefruit Diet, the Banana Diet, the Airline Hostess Diet (I certainly won't be eating any of *them*), the Rice Diet, Fruit Diets, the Martini Olive Diet, the Great Whacking Gobs of Lard Diet. Sorry, I made that last one up. All right, I made the last two up.

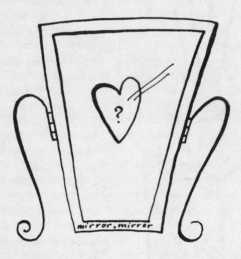

mirror, mirror

Health propaganda In Australia, the National Heart Foundation, well-funded and with a variety of free publications and credibility with the media, is at the forefront of telling people to lose weight and diet. But is it really a sensible angel of mercy or just another part of the anti-fat hysteria?

The Heart Foundation does recommend a long-term, healthy eating plan, with exercise but other attitudes it encourages can be a worry.

The Weight Loss Guide published by the National Heart Foundation has some disturbing messages, including the first section: ways of telling if you are overweight. 'Take off your clothes and stand in front of a mirror. Can you see extra flesh where it shouldn't be? Do parts of your body wobble too much? The mirror doesn't lie. While in front of the mirror try the pinch test. Pinch a good layer of skin over your tummy. If you can pinch more than 2.5 cm you're likely to benefit from losing some body fat.' (The pinch test is rubbish.)

The booklet then recommends the Waist–Hip Ratio and a weight for height chart. The only really sensible test here is the Waist–Hip Ratio, if health is the concern. As for the rest of it, the Heart Foundation does not say how much wobble is all right. Given that all healthy bodies *and* super-lean athletes have wobbly bits, it seems unnecessarily alarmist to suggest that wobbling in itself is a problem at all. There's nothing wrong with the odd wobble, darling. Why do you think belly dancing has been around for thousands of years?

Unfortunately, because of weight-loss propaganda, most women look in the mirror and wrongly believe they have weight 'where it shouldn't be': on their hips and thighs.

And as for the mirror not lying, we know this to be untrue. The mirror is telling porkies. The body-image distortions previously displayed only by those with eating disorders are now experienced by what may be a vast majority of women. Some studies suggest that 80 per cent of women see themselves as larger than they really are.

The first benefit of weight loss suggested by the National Heart Foundation is 'You look better'. The second, 'Feel better about yourself'. The third, 'Look younger'. The fourth, 'Can be more active'. It is not until the fifth reason that health is even mentioned: 'Can lower blood cholesterol, high blood pressure and high blood-glucose levels.'

The British Heart Foundation also recommends the Waist-Hip Ratio test, but their information is much more sensible and geared towards health rather than looks; basically, if you are very overweight, you are more likely to suffer a heart attack.

The diet predators

Even though they know so few succeed in losing weight permanently or even for a significant period, plenty of people are happy to take your money for their diet books or 'programmes'.

> I'm 15 years old and have been on crash diets since I was eleven. But I just can't seem to lose much or last on it long. Being on a diet makes me feel empty and bored. When I talk to my parents they think it's easy to lose weight and aren't interested and I end up upset. Nothing like boredom or stress makes me eat. I just can't help it.
>
> Susie, 15

One magazine sent out undercover investigative reporters to expose the hard-sell tactics used by some diet companies. Luckily for them, clients are usually so humiliated by their sense of dieting 'failure' that they either blame themselves (with some encouragement from popular myths) or are too embarrassed to make a formal complaint.

The weight-loss programmes investigated had misleading advertising, confusing price systems and there were obligations to buy the food marketed by the companies. Customers were asked to sign contracts containing clauses that suggest the companies would not have to fulfil their obligations under the law if a customer was unsatisfied, even though the law actually holds them to such an obligation.

The undercover reporters were told they needed to lose weight but they were not overweight by any health guidelines.

In 1993 a newspaper reporter, rated by a well-known nutritionist as only four and a half pounds heavier than underweight and only nine pounds from dangerously underweight, turned up at several weight-loss centres to check them out. One representative said she should lose the nine pounds. Another employee wanted her to lose a stone to be a 'beautiful size 8'. A toning salon company said almost half a stone should go. Only a Health Solutions Centre told her not to bother and strongly advised her not to go anywhere else.

Genevieve Blais, a British counsellor for people with eating disorders, tells how clients report their 'failure' with weight-watching clubs. They were given ridiculously low target weights that they knew they could never achieve. One client was publicly humiliated when she returned to the club having regained her weight. The speaker made her stand up in front of the group and said 'This is what will happen to you if you don't follow the programme'. How charming.

The cigarette diet Millions of women, who say they want to lose weight to be healthier smoke cigarettes, afraid to give up in case they put on weight. Even the most furious anti-fat lobbyist has to admit that smoking cigarettes is a much greater danger to your health than extra weight.

Diet drugs make you insane Even recommended doses can cause insomnia, crankiness and false levels of energy. Former users report addiction, collapses, hallucinations, malnutrition and the loss of jobs and friends. These pills are 'legalised uppers' as one addict wrote in her account to a magazine. When she came off them 'cold turkey', without help, her heart rate dropped almost enough to kill her.

Appetite suppressants are very dangerous because your appetite is a natural thing. Eating when you're not hungry may be a problem but it's not a great idea to suppress your real hunger. Diet Breakers, an anti-diet group, receives 400 letters a week, many from women who suffered insomnia and dizziness after being prescribed appetite suppressants at slimming clinics. These prescriptions were written by doctors and I'd like to give them a good slapping.

> I'm fat...I'm not overweight for my height but I have stretch marks all over my hips and thighs. I read once in Dolly that if you can pinch more than one inch of fat from your thighs, stomach or underarm, you need toning.* I have tried so many diets. You wouldn't believe how many. Since I turned 14 six months ago I have been on a constant diet. Usually I go for about a fortnight living on virtually nothing (1000 calories a day) and then I can't stand it any more and so I eat whatever I want. And the worst bit is I'm not losing any weight. If you ask me, it sux. It is just not fair. My philosophy is that if you've got a good bod, guys will forgive you for being ugly. Boys like girls who are thin.
>
> Sandra, 15
>
> *Note: the pinch test is not a useful guide to anything.

Other stupid ideas Bulking agents that make you feel full or puff up in your stomach are weird and can be dangerous. Lozenges to deaden taste, sold in chemists, can make your tongue and mouth go numb and must be the ultimate in party-pooper ideas, making it impossible to enjoy food. This in turn encourages you to eat more to get the pleasure you once had.

Liquid diets have killed a few people and spectacularly failed others. This rapid weight loss is almost always followed by rapid weight gain; placing a stress on the body much more dangerous than obesity. *Dolly* magazine warned that liquid diets do not have a long-term effect, make it harder to lose weight, and the sugar level in drinks makes you crave more sugar and food. *Allure* warned against the juice fasting: some US juice companies were suggesting a seven-day fast using their products. The National Institute of Health recommended that no dieter undertake a regime of less than 800 calories a day without medical supervision. The juice diet had ninety.

Fasting is also stupid. I don't care what anybody says about toxins or religious experiences.

Hip and thigh diets, or others claiming to work on one part of the body, are just bizarre. I

> When I was 17 years to 19 years old I was trying diet pills (average of ten a day) and laxatives. Diet pills and medications like it should be prescription only.
>
> Annette, 25

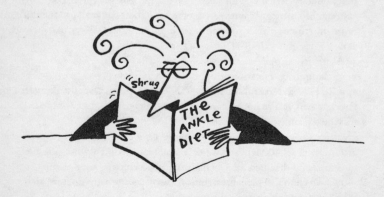

mean, wouldn't you be a teensy bit suspicious of the earlobe diet, or the ankle and left buttock diet? The lose-weight-from-your-knees-and-your-instep diet? 'No, I can't have a cakie thing, I'm trying to lose weight from my wrists.' Get outta here.

'Replacements' A biscuit is not a meal. A small pile of gravel is not a meal. A powdered drink is not a meal. There is almost nothing more than these supplements likely to drive you to eating a real meal or a large buffalo with chocolate fudge cake very soon afterwards. We don't need to replace meals with something else. We need to replace our diet obsession with meals.

Slimmer magazine says, 'The [meal replacement] cookies may be filling (due to their high fibre content) and more nutritious than ordinary biscuits (due to an added vitamin and mineral mix) but they don't re-train your eating habits and they're expensive.'

On another page of the same issue of the magazine it says, strangely, 'Those curves need keeping in check'. Working round to a promotion the magazine continues, 'Limmits Meal replacements are a convenient way to control your calorie intake...they can be used to replace one or two meals during the day, followed by a healthy balanced meal in the evening...Limmits are high in fibre, which makes them pleasantly filling and satisfying [so is sawdust, presumably] helping you to avoid feeling hungry between meals [or meal replacements?] We have 100 samples of Limmits Strawberry Cream biscuits to give to *Slimmer* readers who send their name and address...' And their brain?

Why laxatives do not work Laxatives do not make you lose fat because the nutrients are absorbed before the waste is expelled. The only 'weight loss' is a temporary loss of water.

Tea time The herbal teas usually associated with weight loss are simple diuretics, which only get rid of water. Magazine ads for

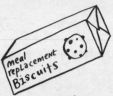 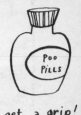

not a meal ...   *not a meal ...*   *not even close ...*   *get a grip!*

Yoland Lim's Oriental Secret go on to reveal that his only secret is having the audacity to claim that his capsules are a seven-day slimming program on which 'you can lose kilograms in the shortest possible time'. The ingredients? Just herbs and vitamins.

The solution There *is* a solution. It means no more hunger, no more expensive foods and supplements you wouldn't normally buy. It does mean you have to be brave and willing to buy fresh food. It means the end of guilt, the end of forbidden foods, the end of food obsession. It means throwing away all the diets and trying to find the time to exercise if you can.

It means *eating whatever you want to*. Aaaaaargh! This is a revolutionary idea and scary for people who crave chocolates and 'bad' foods all the time. But

> Magazine diets usually involve spending money on foods that we don't normally keep around the house, or spending time exercising daily which I'm too lazy to attempt, so I just stay with the cheap and simple starvation diet. The few kilograms I do lose I put straight back on again in a week.
>
> Fran, 19

think about it – maybe the only reason you're so crazy about those foods is that you won't let yourself have them. You have to make friends with your body, live in it and trust it.

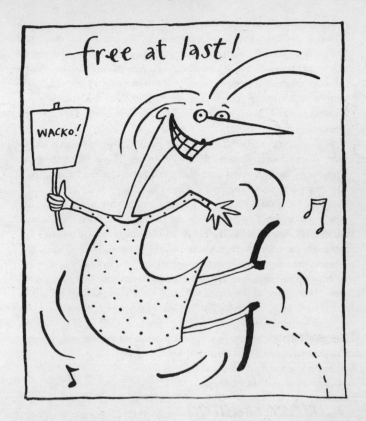

Dr Jane Ogden's theory is that if you take away food restrictions and dieting to lose weight, food becomes less of an obsession, you eat when you need to eat, and your body finds its natural weight. 'There is no need for most people to expect a large weight increase when they stop dieting – their bodies usually find a natural, set weight,' she explains.

Community nurse Penelope Goward agrees: 'Stop dieting and restricting food. We need to give ourselves permission to eat and trust our body's signals. Eat when you are hungry (about every three to five hours) and when you want to. Do not add up any calories or think about the nutritional value of food. Rely on and trust your own body.'

Long-time dieters who have followed this idea in the US are at first a little freaked out by all the permission. Geneen Roth, who runs workshops called Breaking Free, says, 'They think they will eat 12 gallons of icecream and six pizzas and dozens of doughnuts.' When she stopped dieting herself, Geneen Roth at first ate only chocolate chip biscuits and the dough they were made from. She says she was learning what her body was really asking for. She levelled off after the first gain.

When Lauralee Roark, who now runs Beyond Hunger workshops stopped after years of dieting, she said, 'It was like letting the tiger out of the cage. I ate everything that wasn't nailed down...(but) now my body says "broccoli" as loud as it once said "chocolate".' Penelope Goward adds, 'Deal with the underlying issues that cause you to eat when you are not hungry. Attend women's groups or compulsive eating and body image workshops that have an anti-diet approach. Stop discussions about weight control, bodies, diets and weight, and stop complimenting others for weight loss.

'Most of us are not meant to be thin or even slim by today's standards. We're not all the same weight for the same reason we're not all the same height, or same hair colour, or whatever. Accept and like yourself for who you are. Stop postponing your life until you are an acceptable shape and size. Feel good about yourself, for who you are and your unique contributions to life.'

Further reading

Lesléa Newman, *Eating Our Hearts Out* (The Crossing Press, Freedom, California, 1993)

Paulette Maisner with Rosemary Turner, *Consuming Passions: What to Do When Food Rules Your Life* (Thorsons, 1993)

Jasbindar Singh and Pat Rosier, *No Body's Perfect: Dealing with Food Problems* (Attic Press, Dublin, 1990)

Susan Dyson, *A Weight Off Your Mind: How to stop worrying about your body size* (Sheldon Press, 1991)

Dr Tom Sanders and Peter Bazalgette, *You Don't Have to Diet* ▶ (Transworld, 1994)

Obesity

What is obese? Perfectly normal women will wail about being 'fat' or 'obese'. But what does 'obese' mean exactly?

Obesity is defined by some as when a fully developed person is over 30 on the Body Mass Index scale (see page 18). Others say it is being 20 per cent or more above what is considered one's ideal weight range. It is different to being overweight, although the two are often lumped together as if there were no difference.

Who is obese? Obesity seems to be increasing – probably as a result of less exercise and more junk food and fast food, which have high fat and salt contents. According to the British Heart Foundation, we are definitely getting more obese: from 8 per cent of women in 1980 to 15 per cent in 1991, and from 6 per cent of men to 13 per cent over the same period.

One easy way to become obese is to go on a lot of diets. (Sounds crazy? The diets section will explain.)

> I eat breakfast because I have to as Mum makes that every morning, and she makes my lunch every day but I never eat that. I always chuck it in a bin at school. My dinner I usually end up flushing down the toilet, I wait until everyone has left the kitchen, and then head for the toilet and lie to Mum and say I've already eaten. I also drink about two litres of water a day as I heard that water breaks up fat* and makes it easier to lose it. I still get the urge to pig out, say, if I'm depressed and then I end up buying a packet of chocolate biscuits and eat the whole packet. I have reached my goal of being skinnier than my sister. I found out recently that my sister had bulimia.
>
> Julie, 16
>
> *Note: water does not 'break up fat'.

A psychologist from an Eating Disorders Clinic says the clinic found large differences between obese men and women. Men tended to be larger, not worried about their weight and found it easier to lose the weight. Women had a more complex attitude to food – many expected to cook for others but remain slim.

The British Heart Foundation says that in 1990, 47 per cent of men and 45 per cent of women were overweight or obese.

Causes of obesity The most common cause of obesity is overeating and lack of exercise, sometimes for psychological reasons. (Just as undereating, overtalking and underpoliteness and everything else we do is caused by psychological reasons.) 'We live in a society that says fat is bad,' says community health nurse Penelope Goward. 'People panic and start getting obsessed about it and they end up eating more. If we didn't live in a society which suffers from fat phobia, we wouldn't have so many fat people.' She believes many fat people have a good self-image and those who don't, have a bad one imposed by the disapproval of others.

Starting young A dietitian at the Royal Alexandra Hospital for Children in Sydney, Australia, Susan Thompson says, 'If a child has two obese parents he or she has an 80 per cent chance of being obese. Children with two slim parents have a less than 10 per cent chance of being obese. Quite a lot of studies have shown that obesity is genetic rather than environmental...[but] the biggest contributing factors would be a high fat intake, overeating and a lack of activity. Children's activity levels are dropping.' Kids who exercise about as much as a housebrick are at the highest risk.

About 12 per cent of 11 to 16 year olds are overweight (not obese), according to a survey of 700 pupils in Exeter by Dr Neil Armstrong. Dr John Court, director of a Centre for Adolescent Health, told a conference on children's nutrition that parents and teachers should not pressure 'fat' children to lose weight. Genetics made up some of the reasons and lack of exercise was the main problem, he said. 'If you are overweight and that is your constitution then it is not necessarily a health hazard,' Dr Court said. 'Parents must recognise the fact that many overweight children are perfectly normal and should not be constantly subjected to diets that set them up for failure.'

Dr Louise Bauer, a paediatrician, agreed that lack of exercise was the problem but dismissed the tendency for people to think overweight children would 'grow out of it'. She claimed that an overweight adolescent had a 70 to 80 per cent chance of being obese as an adult.

Is it dangerous? Some doctors say obesity is dangerous; others disagree. As far as I can make out over the din of experts fighting about it, being very, very overweight – obese – does carry some health risks. But it also protects from other risks. Being overweight or slightly overweight usually does not carry increased risk of health problems. That is, you can carry around a few extra kilos above your healthy weight range without increasing your risk of anything much except carrying around extra weight.

Anyway, here are the arguments: The National Heart Foundation, which does not like obesity at all, says obese people are twice as likely to die as people in a 'healthy' weight range, and more likely to contract disease, have accidents and commit suicide. Other studies find that obese people are less likely to fall ill than the underweight (see diet section).

It is definitely possible to be fat and healthy. A 'spare tyre' around the middle is dangerous but evenly distributed fat is not necessarily dangerous and, in fact, may mean less health problems than for the underweight.

Real obesity can cause health problems, including diabetes and heart disease. It can be very difficult for obese people to lose weight, partly because of habit and partly because their metabolisms can be very slow. Ironically, some obese people are prone to malnutrition because they eat junk food and do not get enough vitamins and minerals. But obese people do not necessarily eat more than thin people.

Penelope Goward, community health nurse and the head of the Victorian Health Promotion Foundation's Body Image and Eating Behaviour Project in Australia (who must have a very large business card) says, 'Obese people need to be assessed with respect. Not all of them have underlying problems. Sometimes it's just good old genetics and their bodies are adapted to that size. If there are underlying (psychological) issues, they can be worked on,' she says. She recommends that people who think they have a problem with obesity should contact a community health nurse, doctor or counsellor.

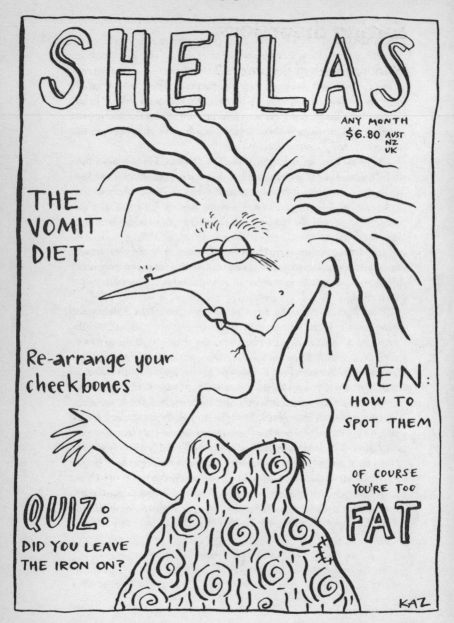

Eating disorders

Who has eating disorders? 'Almost all women do have
an eating disorder,' says a doctor working in the field. 'All the magazines emphasise it and even a book like this will draw attention to
it again…if it were a book for men it would only have one paragraph.
Eating disorders are increasing in men but not as much as they are in
women.'

And now for the statistics. In *Fear of Food*, Genevieve Blais cites the
Royal College of Psychiatrists which says that at least one per cent of
teenage girls suffer from full blown anorexia and another two to three
per cent have partial anorexic syndromes. It is thought that at least
two per cent of women between the ages of 15 and 45 suffer from full
scale bulimia with another four to five per cent of this population
showing partial syndromes. The Eating Disorders Association reck-
ons that the figures are much higher than those reported. It estimates
that up to 200,000 Britons have an eating disorder. The post-1960
girl sees more images of impossibly 'beautiful' women engage in
'sexy' poses in one day than her mother saw through her entire adolescence.

A study of women aged 14 to 25 conducted in Australia in 1983
found that 20 to 30 per cent were bulimic or anorexic, the majority
of them bulimic. Both eating disorders are most prevalent in young
women. The problems usually begin in the teenage years.

Half of teenage girls use extreme dieting ideas to try to lose weight,
according to the 1993 report of an Australian study of 600 adolescent
boys and girls. Extreme weight-loss methods associated with anorexia and bulimia had been tried by 48 per cent of girls and 26 per cent
of boys: at least weekly by 13 per cent of girls and 9 per cent of boys.

A study of 30 bulimic and 30 anorexic patients at the RPH Unit
found that they shared many things, including a dissatisfaction with
their thighs and stomachs. Eighty-three per cent of the bulimic
patients vomited each week (an average of 11.7 times), 33 per cent
abused laxatives, 10 per cent took diet pills. About one-quarter of the
anorexics made themselves vomit on average four times a week.

The mean age at which both groups started worrying about their
weight was about 14 years 7 months. About 15 years 7 months was

the mean age for the onset of dieting and disordered eating behavior. Thirteen per cent of the bulimics had a history of anorexia, and 46 per cent of the anorexics displayed features of bulimia. Sixty per cent of anorexics weighed themselves at least several times a week, but 30 per cent rarely or never did. Fifty to 60 per cent of both groups did not count calories. Only 46 per cent of the anorexia patients admitted they were too thin.

That's a lot of numbers adding up to a lot of sadness.

Most of the definitions and symptoms of anorexia and bulimia presented here are culled from information provided by the RPH Eating Disorders clinic, as well as Health Department information, and books. Not all people with eating disorders are the same, so the symptoms and feelings described are best viewed as tendencies rather than rules.

Anorexia and bulimia can result in a lifetime struggle with the condition, or even death. Long-term emotional problems are believed to be both cause and effect of the disorders, although sufferers and doctors all agree that the social pressures to diet and to be slender can trigger or encourage the conditions.

Many people with anorexia and bulimia have in common a low self-esteem and a cruel perfectionism that allow themselves no flaws in appearance or performance of any activity undertaken. A small flaw – a wrong note in a whole concert, a 98 per cent score – is seen as a failure. 'A significant number of anorexics and bulimics have been victims of rape, molesta-tion and incest,' according to the clinic. Often their families are having problems, sometimes hidden and not admitted to, but many people with eating disorders come from loving families that are healthy and supportive.

— I have binged for three years. I hate it. I hate me. I feel worthless and out of control.
— Good luck.
— For ladies with eating problems; stop watching TV and reading glossy glamour magazines – re-educate the mind and the peace with your body will follow.

Graffiti in University law faculty women's toilets

Many women with eating disorders are in pursuit of happiness which they believe will come if they look thinner.

real *gorgeous*

Anorexia nervosa The girl in the coffee shop having 'lunch' with her friends orders only a glass of water. Her elbows are painfully large compared with her bone-thin arms. Her eyes are shadowed, her hair dull. She says she is not hungry. She is starving.

Anorexia nervosa is a psychological disease that causes a patient to restrict food drastically or not to eat food at all. It is carelessly called a 'slimmer's disease'; actually, it is self-imposed starvation to lose weight. Classic anorexics believe they are heading towards the mythical perfect body as demanded by society, and they believe that by controlling their bodies they are controlling their lives.

One Eating Disorders clinic estimates that each year one in every 200 female teenagers becomes anorexic. The prevalence drops by half in people aged over 17 years. The prognosis can roughly be divided into: 50 per cent recover though 'some may be quirky around food'; 45 per cent have chronic recurrence; 5 per cent die from suicide or heart failure.

The Eating Disorders Association states that anorexia nervosa has 'one of the highest mortality rates of all psychiatric illnesses – over 10 per cent of sufferers die either from the effects of starvation or by committing suicide'.

Anorexics may have abnormal neatness and control about themselves and their environment, and are perfectionists in every project. Their realities tend to be in extremes. Something is either fabulously good or disgusting, beautiful or ugly, fat or thin. Anorexics, and sometimes their families, may deny any problem and resent offers of help.

Classic anorexics often feel that what they think, say and do has little or no impact on other people. Control over their bodies substitutes for control over other parts of their lives. Potential anorexics and bulimics tend to be the 'good children' who please their parents, who presume this means there is nothing wrong with their children. Anorexics are often passive, agreeable children who do not express their own wants and needs and who can eventually rebel by not eating, creating the first major power struggle in the relationship.

Symptoms can include overexercise, vomiting, laxative abuse, diuretics, appetite suppressants, deceitful behaviour to avoid eating ('I ate before'; 'I've had lunch'; 'I'm not hungry'), a relentless pursuit of thinness, covering up the body with baggy clothes, a failure to register what the body really looks like (saying 'I'm fat' when skeletal);

an obsession with food, shape, size in oneself and others. Anorexics often memorise calorie charts, read nutritional books, shop for food and plan elaborate meals they do not eat.

Physical consequences can include loss of periods, weakness, osteoporosis or bone damage, hair loss, pigment changes, skeletal appearance, stunted growth, about a trillion vitamin and mineral deficiencies, starvation, hallucinations and ultimately, for some, death.

> After six months of throwing up I looked terrible, blisters on my knuckles from rubbing against my teeth, broken capillaries around my eyes and swollen glands around my jaw. My skin had broken out in spots and most importantly I was experiencing mood swings and bouts of deep depression. I know the only way out of this is to accept my body at its natural weight. But the trouble is I just can't, and I can't see any way out of this. I just don't know how to relate to food any more. I miss being normal, I envy people who eat and enjoy their food. I live for the day the fuller figure comes back into fashion.
>
> Carrie, 23

According to a doctor at an eating disorders clinic, the best way to help or cure anorexia is to get early recognition and diagnosis of the problem and early intervention. People who have the onset later in life often have a better chance of recovery. Support from friends or family is another crucial factor. A person who has displayed anorexic behaviour for 20 years has less chance of recovery.

'Often these patients have other problems such as a dysfunctional family. Most remember the time they began worrying about their weight. A brother might say she has a big bum: (this) is a common one,' says the doctor. Karen Carpenter, the American singer who died from anorexia, started dieting when a newspaper article described her as 'chubby'. Actress Tracey Gold, ironically from the show *Growing Pains,* was hospitalised with anorexia. She started starving herself when a casting agent made a rude comment about her body.

The doctor adds that, 'Ambitious, achieving girls between 12 and 25 are especially vulnerable. However in industrialised countries the condition is becoming epidemic in all age groups and both sexes.'

Anecdotal evidence suggests that girls at private schools have a higher rate of anorexia. Social worker Julie Dickinson said she believed the pressures to achieve there were more intense. 'The drive

I've had anorexia for about 18 months. Eating disorders are almost always the symptom of a very severe emotional problem, *not* a diet gone wrong. Now I realise that starvation was the only way I felt able to communicate the emotional turmoil inside. I was taken to the cardiac ward...I kept telling them there'd been a mistake there was nothing wrong with me. Mum left in hysterics and I was alone in a strange hospital bed while nurses tried to coax me into eating.

In the middle of the night I was woken by a loud alarm. My heart rate had dropped below 35 beats per minute and technically I was dying. I was transferred to the eating-disorders ward at a private hospital. After my repeated refusals to co-operate I was placed on the dreaded 'program'. Everything was taken

away from me and I was forced to stay in bed in my pyjamas. I had no visitors, no books, phone calls. I had to earn my privileges by weight gain. These attempts to pacify my strong will failed and three weeks later I was transferred again to a medical hospital.

This time it was a real emergency: I was taken in an ambulance complete with oxygen mask and stretcher to the intensive care unit. My spirit was cracked by the private hospital's harsh punishments. I left even more absorbed with food and self-hatred than when I arrived. Since then I have had four hospital admissions and still remain at a very low weight. If what I have said so far is any use to you then it is worth the pain of reflecting on it.

Jane, 16

for high achievement and excellence and the accompanying competitiveness, which are often part of the ethos of independent schools, feed into perfectionism and encourage the view that high achievement is of prime importance and the only way to be valued as a human being,' she said. Bulimia is more evenly spread across state and private schools.

Bulimia nervosa After midnight a silent woman carefully opens the fridge door. She sits alone and stuffs food into herself without pleasure. She gorges on enough for five full meals. She tiptoes to the bathroom, closes the door and puts her fingers down her throat.

Bulimics are trapped in a cycle of binge-eating, guilt and purging. Figures vary as to how many bulimics there are. Most doctors believe that the problem is much more widespread than anorexia but estimations vary from 3.8 per cent to 19 per cent in the US. A 1989 Australian study suggested 1 to 2 per cent of the population. A New Zealand study revealed only a 0.02 per cent rate of bulimia in the general population. Bulimia, some believe, affects one in 100 girls. Over three years with proper treatment 80 per cent improve, 20 per cent persist. Some move to a mixture of anorexia and bulimia.

Bulimia is known to be far more common among teenagers and young women, and more likely in women whose weight is deemed relevant to work or to other pursuits such as ballet, acting, and modelling.

Surveys in schools and colleges have turned up results of 4 per cent and 10 per cent. The problem may be more widespread — bulimia is so secretive it's harder for observers to identify than anorexia.

Bulimics can eat like everybody else but take lots of laxatives to 'purge' the food. They can only do so after kilojoules have been absorbed anyway: most bulimics don't know that the weight loss after laxatives and diuretics is not the food but water loss. Bulimics can seem overweight or underweight.

Their condition is characterised by binge-eating and then purging the food through vomiting, or laxative and diuretic abuse, exercising, dieting, abuse of diet pills and fasting. Binge eating is the fast eating of a large amount of food or almost constant nibbling, associated with a sense of being out of control. Food restriction and dieting are also common and so is depression.

Bulimics can display many of the symptoms of anorexia but while anorexics feel in control of their eating and not much else, bulimics feel totally out of control with eating, in contrast to their high-achieving, well-regulated life. They tend to do their bingeing in secret. Some food is chewed and then spat out. A bulimic often diets, and then has to succumb to the body screaming for carbohydrates, and binges. Then the guilt begins and the cycle continues.

The horrible turmoil is a hidden one. Bulimics tend to be passive people who want attention and approval (who doesn't?). Generally speaking, they have some difficulty in being honest about their needs, and they hide their insecurity and self-doubt behind a busy social life.

Apart from misery, physical consequences can include gastroin-

Next Thursday at 9.30 am I truly face my problem of 12 years. My fiance and I are seeking professional therapy at Prince Alfred Hospital. Bulimia has, to put it bluntly, shot my self-esteem/self-confidence to shit. And yet people are saying how envious they are of me. I bet they wouldn't be that envious if they knew about the anxiety, frustration, self-hatred and depression bulimia has scarred me with. I was vomiting six to eight times a day. These eating disorders are so secretive: you deny black and blue there's anything wrong. Soon after the bulimia took hold I added another 'tool of removal' – laxatives, taking 38 a day (one to two are considered a normal dose). I eventually weaned myself off: being a biologist I know the risks involved. I finally plucked up the courage to tell my fiance – he found it (and still does) very confusing. Now for the psychological battle that begins next Thursday: wish me luck.

Penny, 27

testinal damage, iron deficiency and poor nutrition, diarrhoea, kidney damage from the diuretic pills, a swollen face, calluses on the hand used to induce vomiting, damage to teeth, mouth and gullet from stomach acids, fatal stomach rupture or heart attack. The director of an eating disorders clinic says up to half the patients she has seen with bulimia have previously had anorexia.

Dr Suzanne Abraham of Sydney University and co-author of a book about eating disorders says that with counselling and nutrition, most eating disorder patients recover completely. At last, some good news! 'But it takes a while to get better,' she adds.

Many bulimics can learn how to express their feelings in ways other than those involving food. They learn that they have needs and wants that cannot be met with food, but can be identified and met by other 'rewards' in life.

Training for an eating disorder Although common features of women with eating disorders include their unreal expectations of perfection and difficulty in accepting natural weight gains in the teenage years, that doesn't mean that all ambitious high achievers are anorexics or bulimics. But every authority on eating disorders says parents and teachers should not pressure students to unrealistic goals or to perfection.

What then, to make of the special programme started at a primary school in Sydney where girls, between six and 12 years old, have been chosen to attend a special gymnastics school to prepare them for the Olympics in the year 2000? According to a report in the *Sydney Morning Herald*, the girls will be 'kept together with their teacher...while they are groomed to be great athletes'. Leanne Schmidt, the girls' teacher and a former gymnast, said she did not go through puberty until she was 18-and-a-half, when she stopped training and grew almost 30 centimetres in three months.

Here are little girls who will be taught that becoming a woman, getting periods and the change in body shape is their enemy; to be unnaturally stunted is good and that the definition of their success will be measured by whether they become Olympians.

Even if the girls do not develop eating disorders, how will this delaying of puberty affect them? Can you imagine the outcry if a school announced that it was gathering a team of 12 young boys, aged six to 12, delaying the boys' natural development until they were 18 to keep their voices high so they could sing soprano and be the right height as a special choir to sing at the opening of the 2000 Olympics?

The Australian Institute of Sport's own psychologist, Jeff Bond, said in 1992 that he believed dozens of Australia's top athletes were suffering anorexia and bulimia. 'I'm talking about the national and international level,' he said.

Mr Bond said, 'There is a much, much stronger emphasis almost year by year now on power-to-weight ratios and low body fat and so on.' He told the *Sydney Morning Herald* that anorexia tended to be a feature of distance and artistic sports such as gymnastics, but bulimia was more prevalent across the board.

I asked Mr Bond about the school for gymnasts, the delaying of puberty for gymnasts and whether this was acceptable policy. He said, 'It's inevitable, I'm not sure it's acceptable. As a parent, as a humanist I'd say it's not acceptable. As a realist, working within the system of elite sport, we (the sports psychologists) try to cushion it as best we can.'

Mr Bond said the stopping of periods through stress from training,

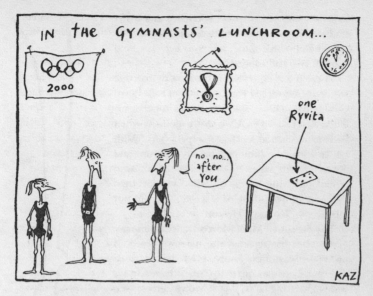

as well as lowered body fat, was 'an accepted thing in elite sport'.

Mr Bond said as a psychologist within the system, he worked to try and make athletes aware that they were just going through a phase in their lives, making great sacrifices, and that they would move on to another phase. He said sometimes the athletes were not aware of all the sacrifices they were making. (I would say that is particularly true for a six-year-old girl enrolled in a gymnasts' school.)

When you watch the Olympics in the year 2000, think of what those little girls have been put through, paid for with Government money.

Ballet According to professor of Psychiatry Peter Beumont, there is evidence that ballet dancers are particularly prone to developing anorexia and bulimia nervosa. He says, 'Their ballet teachers ask them to keep weight levels which are physiologically abnormal. There's a lot of unhappiness amongst many health professionals about the poor advice that many ballet teachers give their students.' Ballet teacher Virginia Gallagher says she guards against the problem with her students because of her own experience as a ballet student. She was given amphetamines and developed bulimia like three others in her class; and another two had anorexia.

There is a long tradition of these destructive requirements. Gelsey Kirkland, one of ballet guru George Balanchine's students, recalls in her autobiography, *Dancing on My Grave*, a moment when Ballanchine halted a class to inspect her. 'With his knuckles, he thumped on my sternum and down my rib cage, clucking his tongue and remarking "Must see the bones". I was less than 100 pounds even then,' she wrote. 'He did not merely say "Eat less". He said "eat nothing!"'

The acclaimed Mark Morris Dance Company of America has rejected the narrow ideal and shows the way of the future. It has dancers of all different shapes and sizes. '[Critics] have always said we have big butts,' Mark Morris agrees. 'We have big butts. The point is: who CARES.'

Modelling Penelope Tree, one of the original 'waif' models from the 1960s, was anorexic as a famous model. She says she started dieting at boarding school because she felt emotionally abandoned. She was 36 before she got bulimia under control. She identifies 'the sad and pitiful irony of beautiful models in beautiful expensive magazines who are destroying themselves for other people'.

She remains convinced that having an eating disorder is rewarded by society. It is seen as glamorous, enviable, professionally successful and financially rewarding for models and actors. She believes that women are trapped into being thinner for other women as part of the competition and that the industry which encourages the unre-

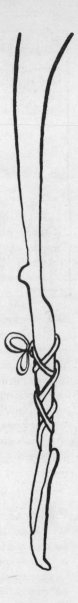

al thinness is bigger than all of us. 'But steps can be taken on an individual basis,' she says. 'Young women, especially adolescents, have to be taught how to feel good about themselves. You have to find something worthwhile to fill the hole of emptiness and confusion that confronts us all when we are growing up.'

Role models Several observers say that a major contributing factor to eating disorders is the widening gap between reality and the cultural ideal. Psychiatrist Dr Jerome Gelb wrote to a newspaper saying he could not 'remain silent while ever-increasing numbers' of young women are referred to him for therapy for their eating disorders. 'Surely it is time for those responsible for influencing our young women and for setting the so-called "ideal" to demonstrate some responsibility and encourage the use of more normal representatives of the female community to sell fashion…It is with great alarm that I have noticed the fashion industry's recent move towards promoting the image of the undernourished, "waif-like gamine" as the latest pinnacle of perfection for women.'

Dr Gelb linked these cultural pressures to the women with eating disorders.

Schoolgirls Jacqueline McArthur and Caitlin MacLeod also wrote to the newspaper, saying 'Lining our walls are *Elle* cutouts of often adolescent *boys* stylised and photographed in women's clothing to shape the unattainable ideal in

> My bulimia has worsened over the past year and I have been in hospital once. Most of the time I feel like a big fat loser because I don't know many winners who stand over the washbasin four or five times a day with their hand down their throat. I know taking laxatives weakens your heart and diet pills dull your brain but if they worked I'd still be taking them. My circulation is stuffed, my face and throat are always puffy, my skin always blotchy and I have broken capillaries from having my head down too often, not to mention scars on my right hand's first two knuckles. Sorry about the pleasant description but the point I'm trying to get across (even to myself) is that bulimia is a dead end. I look even further from the models I was trying to emulate at the start.
>
> Pamela, 17

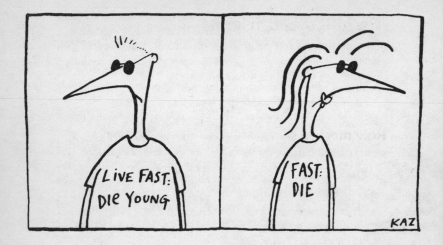

our minds. The toilets no longer smell of smoke, but of vomit. Last year a girl was hospitalised with anorexia nervosa, only to appear six months later gracing the pages of *Dolly* magazine.'

The editor of *Vogue,* Alexandra Shulman, defended her use of waif models by saying, 'I don't understand the fuss. It has been proved over and over again that anorexia and bulimia have nothing to do with fashion pictures. Models have always been thin. Kate Moss is shorter than most models, but no thinner.' That last sentence is laughable to anyone who has seen pictures of Kate Moss. But perhaps it is too easy for Ms Shulman to say that fashion pictures do not cause anorexia and bulimia. They are, at least according to the evidence of many young women struggling with eating disorders and their doctors and therapists, part of their problem.

Several eating-disorder clinics will not allow any women's magazines on the premises.

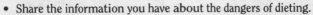

Families and friends

One Eating Disorders clinic suggests the following for friends and parents to help prevent anorexia and bulimia:

- Share the information you have about the dangers of dieting.
- Help others to understand the purposes of advertising images, and why they must not be taken to heart.
- Do not push children or friends to excel in sports and other areas.
- Examine your own motives for wanting those associated with you to excel.
- Adolescents need a mix of rules and freedoms in their lives, without being overprotected or abandoned to fend for themselves. Let friends and children work through their pain and problems by themselves, with your support. Your role is to love, support and encourage. Help young people to understand the difference between a good diet (nutrition) and dieting. Avoid encouraging young people to lose weight.
- Be a good role model for other women. Avoid criticising your own body. Stop talking about physical appearance and diets. Express admiration for healthy bodies, even if they are not thin.
- Be a good role model for other men by not criticising women who do not meet your standards of physical beauty. Don't encourage your wife, girlfriend, sister or daughter to lose weight because you think it would make *you* feel better.
- Talk to friends and children about why they want to lose weight. If it is because of feelings of inadequacy, deal with those issues. If the feelings continue, find a counsellor who is trained to work with eating disorders. The Eating Disorders Association has more information for family and friends.

Getting help

Because the psychological reasons for eating disorders can be so ingrained, many people who have had anorexia and bulimia have relapses and need further help throughout their lives. Others may want to head off the problem before it gets too much.

A range of treatments is available for each disorder, including group

I am 24 years old and have been bulemic [sic] for approximately six to seven years. I was anorexic at 48 kilos (seven and a half stone). I was running the family home at 11 and sexually abused by my uncle at three years old and I was always a fat child. I remembered when I was twenty-one. My mother and sister were both models: I was acknowledged for being clever but ugly. Nearly every girl I know has or has had an eating disorder: three bulimic, one anorexic, three bulimic and anorexic, one obese and four normal. It appears the younger girls are the more prone to disorders. My older friends have grown up with less pressure or have just learned to accept their bodies the way they are.

Rula

therapy, psychotherapy and counselling, nutritional counselling, assertion training, family therapy, and hospitalisation only in very severe cases.

People may take time to find the right therapist. One ex-bulimic encourages those who need help not to be discouraged if the first doctor or psychiatrist doesn't understand the problem or is contemptuous of it. It is very important that you contact an anorexia and bulimia support group so you can talk to people who really understand and will not judge you. Contact the British Associaton for Counselling for further information.

Many people have been cured of their eating disorders, others have their eating disorders as background to their lives, but manageable. Many are particularly helped by making the decision to go to therapy – not as a failure but as a positive step to helping themselves and becoming well, a new challenge.

Don't go to a therapist who offers you quick cures or a better cure for more money or those who talk only of willpower or do not see the problem as serious. Therapists can have their own problems and biases.

Bulimia is a struggle every day. In the end it gets me nowhere: I have achieved no significant weight loss from this. This eating disorder is caused mostly by my desire to be thinner but after thinking it over I've discovered that in a small way it is also attributed to my need for more attention because I live in a large family where there isn't a lot of attention to go around.

Haylie, 19

Laxatives make ya bum sting.

Georgina, 15

Many experts recommend the best place to start is your local doctor. Ask for a full examination and if necessary, referral to an eating-disorders clinic. If you feel too heavy or too light, seek help or information. Most women are treated as private patients or people who visit the hospital but don't have to stay there.

Your local doctor may not be experienced in treating eating disorders but can refer you for help or get instructions on how to help you. Nutritionists at eating-disorders clinics and women's health centres can also help you.

The Eating Disorders Association can send you information, give advice over the phone and refer you for further help. You may be surprised to find so many people who share your experiences.

Several private psychiatrists are working in the field of eating disorders. Some of them have personal theories about the causes of anorexia or bulimia which they explore during sessions. While some of these therapists may be very helpful for some women, they are generally not able to help with nutritional advice and programs.

As the causes of the disorders are multi-dimensional, so may be the treatments.

People with eating disorders can feel alone in the wilderness. Actually the wilderness is pretty crowded these days. You can learn to read the signs – especially the ones which say 'Wrong way: go back!'

When asking bulimics to define bulimia, the replies were all associated with feelings, or the effects bulimia had on their lives. Vomiting and laxative abuse were not mentioned...
(comments include)
— It's not living, just existing.
— If you are not doing it, you are thinking about doing it.
— It stops you from living and appreciating the moment. It is paralysing fear.
— Chaotic, not living.
— It blocks out life, it's not living.
— My personal definition of bulimia is when a person's relation to food becomes the medium used in which to express repressed thoughts and feelings.

Lui Suit, bulimia research project

Contacts

Support groups which will send you information or help you on the phone:

Eating Disorders Association
Sackville Place
44 Magdalen Street
Norwich
Norfolk
NR3 1 JU
Helpline 01603 621414
Youth Helpline 01603 765050
Fax 01603 664915

British Association for Counselling
1 Regent Place
Rugby
Warwickshire
CV21 2PJ
Information Line 01788 578328
Office 01788 550899
Fax 01788 562189

Diet Breakers
Church Cottage
Barford St Michael
Banbury
Oxon
OX15 0UA
Phone 01869 37070

A national campaigning organisation looking at the personal, political and social aspects of dieting. It has a holistic approach, helping participants to set realistic, achievable and sustainable goals, starting with self-acceptance and a healthy lifestyle. It is particularly useful for compulsive eaters, obese people and chronic dieters.

Overeaters Anonymous of Great Britain
P.O. Box 19
Stretford
Manchester
M32 1EB
Phone 0171 498 5505

Support group for overeaters

Women's Nutritional Advisory Service
P.O. Box 268
Lewes
BN7 2QN
Phone 01273 487576

Provides an advisory service, which is 'diet-based' for women suffering from PMS and menopausal symptoms, and chocolate/sugar cravings.

Further reading

Jane Hirschmann and Carol Munter, *Overcoming Overeating: Conquer Your Obsession with Food* (Mandarin, 1990)

Genevieve Blais, *Fear of Food* (Bloomsbury, 1995)

Barbara French, *Coping with Bulimia: The Binge/Purge Syndrome* (2nd edn, Thorsons, 1994)

Maroushka Monro, *Talking About Anorexia: How to Cope Without Starving* (Sheldon Press, 1992)

Susie Orbach, *Hunger Strike* (Penguin Books, 1993)

Duker and Slade, *Anorexia and Bulimia: How to Help* (Oxford University Press, 1988)

French, *Coping With Bulimia* (Thorsons, 1994)

Exercise

Too little A 1993 survey of schoolchildren showed that only 5 per cent of girls and only 35 per cent of boys could complete 100 sit-ups in five minutes.

While I have to agree that the survey's other findings were depressing (one-third of girls between 12 and 15 were reportedly 'obese'), is doing 100 sit-ups in five minutes necessarily a desirable or even a sensible thing?

According to the British Heart Foundation, only 10 per cent of men and 3 per cent of women meet the recommended level of physical activity. We're a proud pile of lazy, TV-watching slugs.

Anyway, figures show more unfit girls than boys, and too many girls are being discouraged from sport. They get less recognition, support and funding than boys for their achievement and effort. Which is a complete rip-off, because girls who don't play sport are often less healthy, less confident, and don't like themselves as much as girls who do.

We are up against it here, when less than 5 per cent of newspapers' sports pages are devoted to women's sport. In the last Olympics there were 159 men's events and 86 women's events. Among registered sporting participants, women are outnumbered by men by more than three to one. By their early 20s, so many women have dropped out of sport that the ratio is already 2:1.

In 1989, 33 per cent of women and 51 per cent of men participated in sport. Women were mainly represented in only two sports – tennis and netball. Sixty-five per cent of female students and 81 per cent of male students participated in sport. Between the ages of 15 and 24, three-quarters of women do some exercise.

After that, the numbers drop drastically, and people tend to turn to useless dieting: between the ages of 25 and 34 is the peak time for dieting rather than exercising to lose weight. This is also the time many women are looking after children and possibly working outside the home as well, so finding time for exercise is difficult. While 38 per cent of women said they didn't like sport, another 35 per cent said they had no time, especially mothers.

On average, girls tend to be less effective than boys in some sporting skills such as throwing balls. There is no physical explanation for this. It is about girls being encouraged and taught the same way. And

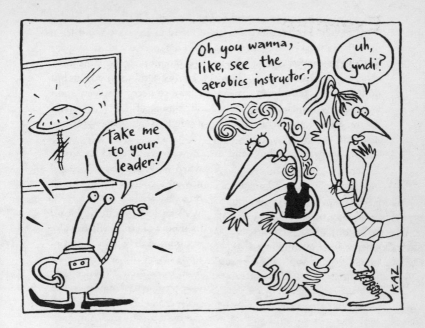

the aerobic fitness (heart-lung working capacity) of girls starts declining, on average, after the age of twelve. Which, *not* coincidentally, is the same age that self-esteem generally starts to plummet through the floor.

According to the Heart Foundation girls are more likely to underrate their performance than boys. If a girl and a boy throw a ball exactly the same distance, the boy is more likely to say, 'That was great', and the girl will think 'Not good enough, I shall go and attempt to drown myself in the science laboratory'. Once they stop, girls seem to get shyer about starting again, being seen by others to make mistakes, and their bodies being seen by others, particularly their new, unfamiliar bodies with breasts and hips. (This is not helped by the taunts of other girls and boys, who are made frenzied and nasty by their own puberty freakouts.)

Girls tend to see sport as a participation, affiliation with others, and a team activity; boys tend to see it more as achievement-based, a view more richly rewarded in the past.

We have to be more like the boys if we're going to get in there and enjoy ourselves. Girls tend not to participate if their skill level is low, whereas boys are braver, more likely to have a go and learn from their mistakes. We have to demand the space we need, as space and equipment for girls to play sport is often much less than those allocated for boys – in schools which are not allowed to do this but do it anyway. This doesn't mean we have to necessarily play sport *with* the boys, which can be a torrid and bruising affair, but we should get the same equipment to, ahem, if you'll excuse the expression, play with ourselves.

We can learn from boys and men how to get up and keep going when we've scraped a knee and missed a goal (without taking on angry feelings at ourselves). We can learn from boys and men how to go on when we're not immediately good at something. Actually we can learn from some men's leagues how to go on when we're never really good at something. We can do it for the fun of it, even if you never hit the top of the ladder.

> I think that magazines for teenagers should have a complete lift-out on what exercises to do for the different parts of the body where people want to lose weight…hips, legs, stomach. I dislike my hips, bum and thighs, they all need a good workout. I look in all the mags and I wish I looked like the models but life goes on!
>
> 'Keen', 13

And maybe some could learn from us that exercising doesn't always have to be only about winning. There's belly-dancing, basketball strategy meetings, archery and long walks looking at the world and taking time out to smell the roses, as long as we don't get thorns up our nostrils.

Too much Too much exercise can encourage some people to become anorexic. Professor of Psychiatry Peter Beumont says that once a person's weight falls below a certain level, behaviour patterns become obvious – the overexerciser stops eating, the overdieter starts exercising.

The professor noted that the overexercisers began their regime because they were concerned about their weight and shape, whereas many anorexics stopped eating properly because of anxiety and other problems.

One kind of overactivity, he said, 'followed too literally the advice of magazines that suggested "never sit if you can stand, never stand if you can walk, never walk if you can run" '. Sufferers of this disorder sometimes get into a complicated, endless 'debt' system, where they eat to reward themselves for exercising, but exercise to punish the eating. This can lead to overexercising anorexia patients being finally admitted to hospital or other treatment in a far worse state than those who were not exercising as well as starving.

(One of the things about exercising is that if you wear polyester hot-pink tights for hours on a stationery cycle you will probably get raging thrush over half of your body, but yet another thing is that if you exercise, you will also have to eat extra protein, iron, calcium and carbohydrates and drink a lot of water.)

Some women look at those charts which tell you how much energy you have to expend to 'lose' some food you've eaten. This is often expressed thus: 'One carrot. Must run around the house for four days and then cycle 200 miles.' Forget these stupid, STUPID charts, which completely ignore the fact that we need the food to make our bodies like, you know, work? Every piece of food you eat is used by the body to make the skin system work, help pump the blood around and replace cells and walk and talk and grow hair. Food has work to do. The equation of eat it and be punished or eat it and then work it off is just crazy. If you see one of these charts, do not approach it; it may be charming and dangerous. Cut it out and feed it to the dog.

Former middle-distance runner Michelle Baumgartner recalls that her strict dieting and athletic training stopped her menstruating at nineteen. At her peak of athletic success her body fat was an astonishing 8 per cent; women should be 22 to 30 per cent. 'It took me five years from the time I stopped training to recover,' she said. 'I suffered from all sorts of problems but my coach and people around would tell me that I looked great and to keep pushing myself...I was underweight and sick and nobody seemed to notice. But if I didn't win it was my fault...[we used to joke] how fantastic it was we didn't have to go through periods. I now realise I was lucky to retire when I did.' Another former running mate had four bone grafts before she was 26 to try and correct the problems.

Overexercise can thin the bones, just as anorexia does, making the body vulnerable to osteoporosis. Some young female athletes are left with the chalky, brittle bones of women in their seventies or eighties. Under intense pressures, female athletes lose a lot of weight, developing eating disorders, stress fractures, menstrual disorders and osteoporosis.

High-impact aerobics and other exercise on a hard surface can cause jarring of joints, tearing of tissue and damage to the inner ear.

Another big drawback of exercise is that it has spawned a repulsive and often risky mountain of celebrity exercise videos by every white-grinned thin movie star, rock star and model with advice from often dubious 'personal trainers' (torturers) focusing on bits of the body – stomach, bottom, hips, thighs. These videos can damage your body, and following their regime can have very little to do with real fitness.

Anyway isn't it a bit lonely, just you and a video?

This is related to the Scary Gyms Full Of Scary People Syndrome – intimidating men with unnaturally wide necks who smell like chemicals when they sweat (that'll be your steroids) and underfed women who look at you strangely if you have legs bigger than breadsticks especially if you're wearing footy shorts and a shape-challenged T-shirt which says 'Pre-Menstrual As Anything'. Some gyms cater for people who are not muscle-bound or vampirical.

> For the last two years I've been doing 100 sit-ups, give or take 50, at least five nights a week, but my weight hasn't changed once. I can't stand it.
> I've come to realise it's mainly got to do with genetics. My parents are heavily built but still healthy.
>
> Mardi, 17

Jane Fonda's multi-million dollar series of 'workout videos' was described as dangerous by some critics, and later it turned out Ms Fonda was bulimic through the whole thing – not a condition that comes under the heading of fitness.

The obsession with exercise has spawned some very stupid marketing ideas: *Allure* magazine says we should wear waterproof make-up while sweating (bad idea). A model used to illustrate the magazine's special on exercise looks to be either extraordinarily naturally thin and bony or else the victim of an eating or exercising disorder: you can see the outline of her bones underneath her skin. The

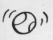

caption reads, 'Fat chance. Sure, low-intensity is just as good as high-intensity exercise – but you have to do it longer.' There is a make-up credit but we cannot see the model's face.

You know those exercises you see in magazines with a maniacally grinning instructor demonstrating each one, or a drawing of a woman who in real life would be nine feet tall and weigh as much as a pocket packet of tissues? You're better off going to an aerobics class with a qualified, sensible teacher or a low-key yoga instructor to show you exactly the right way to do them. Otherwise you may wrench something, or topple over, or just generally make a dork of yourself doing six months of exercises that don't actually exercise anything except your time. Or you could hurt yourself if you develop a bad habit in your own lounge room, such as bouncing on a stretching movement or watching American sitcoms with 'family values'.

Many of these exercises in magazines concentrate on one area of your body, usually thighs, bottom and stomach but sometimes other bits (arms, even). This kind of obsession with one area of the body encourages you to think weirdly about yourself. People will greet you, 'Hi, Jane', and you will say, 'Say hello to my biceps, too, they get lonely'. And doing those sorts of exercises takes time and leaves the other bits to get mouldy and neglected.

Enough It is generally accepted that we would all feel better about ourselves and be healthier if we exercised three times a week. Each time, the exercise should have us breathing much faster than normal for at least 20 minutes, and 40 minutes if possible. Beginners should work up to these levels over time.

Why exercise? Exercise reduces stress and tiredness. Also, you can stop when it hurts, which is more than you can say for life in general. Also, you can choose the best kind for you. This means that if walking up and down three stairs at the gym is boring you until you want to shriek, shriek, *shriek,* you can go and learn the Lambada next door.

It means that if you can't get the motivation to go and interact with a machine three times a week, you can join a team and play sport with humanoids. Exercise makes you more aware of your own body and think of yourself more as a whole being than a collection of parts, or a brain followed around by all that baggage underneath.

The National Heart Foundation, which is always banging on about getting more exercise lists several benefits including improved concentration, relaxation, less tension, sleeping better, improved posture, strength, fitness, improved digestion and easier breathing, greater confidence, feeling happy and relaxed, a healthier blood cholesterol level, lower blood pressure, stronger bones, longer life and less likelihood of a heart attack. Well, that's a bonus.

There are less obvious benefits, such as developing friendships and work contacts through sport; opportunities to learn how to deal with success and failure and a whole lot of other gobbledegook about personal challenges and team efforts and stuff that kind of makes me sick so I won't bore you with it.

Getting started It is extremely hard to get motivated, unless you're like Madonna and have a personal trainer, which is just like hiring somebody to shout at you 'Get up, you lazy dugong!' and then run around after thinking up other insults and saying, 'Hup two three four,' until you strangle them with something made of lycra and get off on justifiable homicide and *still* have to pay them £50 an hour. Anyway, other than that, you may, like somebody I know not entirely unadjacent to *me,* rather lie in bed and see how the dream ends. Or lie in bed and not see how the dream ends. But, basically, for whatever reason seems closest to hand at the time, lie in bed.

Some ways to get around this motivational problem include: paying gym membership in advance (this rarely works, you just lose your money and feel cross with yourself for not going); making a time to walk, run or swim with friends, and playing a team sport so you are in a group that relies on each other to turn up for training and matches.

Another problem with exercise is that if you've never done any, and you suddenly start doing a great deal of it, your body can become totally affronted, and you might die. The way to avoid this is to lead

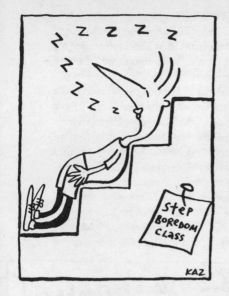

your body into the subject very gently so it hardly gets huffy at all, and before it knows it, it's having its fingertips introduced to the toes and the blood is pumping around, heartily making itself acquainted with all the extremities.

Another drawback of suddenly beginning to exercise can be injury. This can be avoided by kitting yourself out correctly, with the right shoesies and things and, if circumstances require, helmets, kneepads, mouthguards, private health insurance and an ambulance at the bottom of the hill.

You can also avoid injury by not playing the more brutal sports in which skill is less important than the level of truly innovative violence and opportunities for spinal injury and blindness. These include one of the codes of rugby, I can't remember which one, but it's probably the one in which they gaffer tape their ears to their heads in case they get ripped off, and also low-grade ice hockey, and any game in which the opposition has expressed an interest in examining your entrails.

There is quite a lot of sexism in sport, which discourages women from participating and pushes them into early spectatorhood. Part of this is an uneven distribution of funds to sport by schools, governments and sponsors. Another is that girls have been less encouraged to do daring things. In the past, boys were supposed to do strong, exhibitionist, dangerous things (weight-lifting, football), and girls were supposed to do flouncy, pretty things (gymnas-

We interviewed Jamie Lee Curtis who was meant to have the 'perfect body'. She worked out four hours a day for that body. Now she has a child and better things to do with herself.

Diane Parks,
Slimming magazine

tics, ballet). This is changing, and champion girl and women surfers, in-line skaters, cricketers, martial artists, netballers, runners, jumpers, basketballers, soccer players and their sisters in all codes are waiting for you to join them. Just make sure you're fit enough to run if any of them ask to see your entrails.

But we can fight the discrimination and discouragement, and get out there and get the benefits. (Some trumpet music here, please.) Even though women form a smaller part of the Australian Olympic team than men, they have always won more medals proportionately. And we don't even have to be Olympians. We don't even have to want to. I certainly don't – those opening ceremony uniforms are usually embarrassing. (Whoops, sorry, I just channelled the fashion police.)

If you are discriminated against because you cannot use the facilities of a sporting club – whether it's a soccer club or a bowls club, or you're forced to be an associate member, or you're not being given access to equipment at school, you can lodge a complaint, or

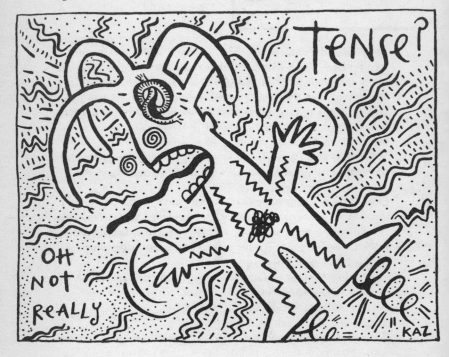

ring for help from the Citizens Advice Bureaux.

You may not choose the right exercise genre first time. In fact it would be amazing if you did not have to try out a few things to see what you liked best. The second time I tried aerobics it was an Afro-Brazilian class where the teacher Mistress Maria played Yothu Yindi (and who would dare to explain to Mistress Maria that Arnhem Land was not in Africa, or even Brazil, but Australia?) and set a literally blistering pace which involved exhorting the class to do things like: 'Now, in time to the music, place your left ankle over your right shoulder and leave it in the far corner of the gymnasium. Now do 800 push-ups. Maybe 900. I don't know yet.'

(A word of warning. Golf. Golf is exercise and golf is stupid. Do not let this put you off exercise itself.)

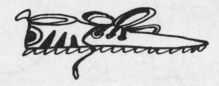

Types of exercise **Aerobic exercise** Lifts your heart
rate, and makes you sweat and breathe quicker. This means stuff like jogging, walking quickly, riding a bike, skipping, aerobics, aquarobics, running around a sports field without stopping and fleeing from a house where they are playing Barry Manilow songs.

Isometric exercise Weight training, often on machines, using small groups of muscles at a time.

Just stuff Walking home from the bus, answering the telephone, ironing, shopping, hanging out the washing, lifting kids, chasing kids, cooking, gardening, using the stairs, living. This actually takes up most of our body fuel: it is the bulk of our energy expenditure.

Vigorous relaxing A more Eastern approach emphasising balance, economy of motion, centring and harmonious use of the body, e.g. yoga, tai-chi, martial arts.

Energetic exercise Abandoned sex and wild dancing.

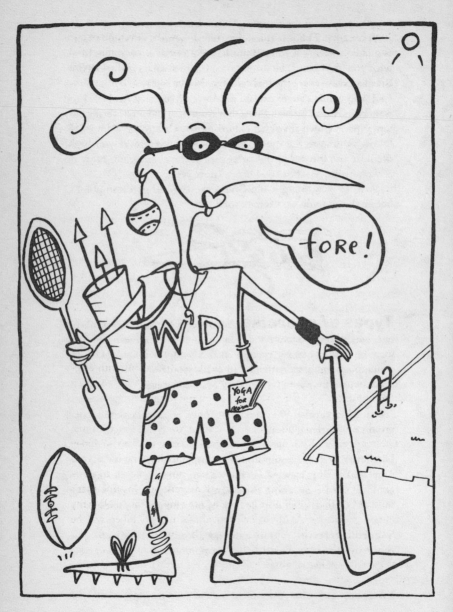

Guru exercise This is when you slavishly follow the directions of one instructor or discipline. Don't forget you can keep an open mind and choose the best bits from anywhere you like. This is called Buffet Exercise. No it's not, I just made that up. Maybe I should have a video.

Simple calorie burning This determined, compulsive exercise is aimed only at losing weight, instead of using all parts of the body and warming up or warming down. Often people who do this look kind of frenzied and desperate.

Fun Things you do with friends, or relatives, or the dog. Frisbee, chatting while walking with a friend, splashing around with an old canoe, learning country-and-western dancing; anything involving a 'hit and giggle'.

Pretendy exercise This is where they strap you to a table and it moves your body for you. Or using those little electrode pads which are taped to your thighs and stomach which are supposed to shape, sculpt or tone your body, according to the brochures. What they do is send little electric impulses into your body. There is usually also a lot of guff about microsecond pulses, monophasic wave forms and longitudinal padding of the muscle. It's a gimmick that claims to 'condition' your body's muscles by jiggling them about with electronic impulses. Often billed as some sort of workout on a couch, it is no substitute for exercise and does nothing for heart-lung fitness.

Avoid exercising which divorces you from yourself (bear with me, I'm not going all New Age hippy on you). Choose an exercise thingy (I hesitate to use the word plan. I have always hesitated to use a word like plan, and I'm sorry but I just can't start now)...choose an exercise thingy that's fun, that's about *you* exercising. Not one that's about: 'My right thigh is now exercising; now my left thigh. Now my bum is exercising. At about half-past three, my left bicep will be distinguishing itself.' Also, do *not* weigh yourself and freak out. Muscle weighs more than fat. It doesn't mean you're overweight. Anyway, you know what you should do with bathroom scales. Sledgehammers ahoy!

Beware of exercise and jargon that encourages body hatred, or sees the body as the enemy. So avoid 'bottom burners', 'stomach crunchers' and such careless nasty talk about yourself.

The very best magical thing about exercising

I will admit that exercise does have one perfectly magical effect. It makes you feel better about yourself. It makes you feel good about yourself. Exercise, if I could just make things utterly clear, raises your self esteem. Just about any form of exercise will do this except one where you're surrounded with neurotic people in mauve leotards who are comparing people's body shapes and making you feel inadequate so they can feel better about themselves, or except when the main reason for exercise is that your body is seen as the enemy: 'I have to get rid of these hips.'

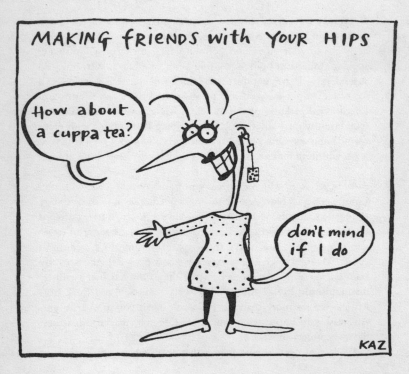

And this feeling better about yourself happens *regardless* of your weight or shape. If you're a size 16 and you exercise regularly and you are meant to be size 16 and you stay a size 16, you will *like yourself more*.

This is the one truly fabulous thing about exercise, and it is just a great shame that it is not really something you can do while you are asleep.

Further information

The British Heart Foundation has enough information on all this stuff to choke a shire horse, and they have free pamphlets to send to individuals and schools.

Your local council will have a list of activities and classes such as yoga, dance and aerobics. Ask about the qualifications of your instructor.

Your council will also have information about sporting groups in the area. You can join by yourself, or with a friend.

Check out your local sports clubs. Many are gathering points for organised walking or other activities.

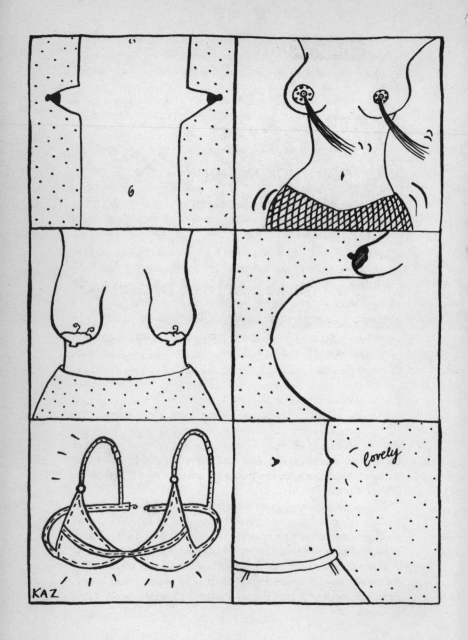

chapter *three*

What is normal?

Do I have normal breasts?

32B or not 32B Unless you have breasts shaped like question marks, they're probably normal. Most women have a right breast larger than their left. Just about everyone will develop stretch marks with their first breast growth spurt. Later, hairs will grow around the nipple. Normal breasts can be very small or very large (girls and women with larger breasts can have neck, chest and back pain from bra straps holding the weight and suffer cruel comments and rude stares).

These women at the outer edge of the normal range can find it difficult to get bras to fit them – not because they're not 'normal' but because the manufacturers don't make the same profits from the women who ask for a bra size they don't sell the most of: 32B or not 32B, that is their question.

Breasts are for feeling good when they're touched and for breastfeeding, whatever their size. Small breasts may be easier for breastfeeding because there is less to get in the way when a baby is suckling. Breastfeeding provides natural immunities against sickness for a baby, as well as being its only food in the early months. After breastfeeding the breasts may be smaller and less outwardly pointing than before. With age, especially after the menopause, the breasts become less plumped out.

> My breasts often seem too small.
>
> Fran, 19
>
> I'm as flat as a pancake. All the other girls my age have breasts and I don't. It's very embarrassing. PS: How do you get into this modelling business?
>
> Judy, 13

Breasts can be round, hard, soft, lumpy, irregularly shaped, shaped like test tubes, large, small, shaped like quinces, shaped like ferret noses, pointed in opposite directions, high, low, bounce from side to side or up and down, with cleavage, far apart, with freckles, with pink nipples and areola (the coloured area around the protruding nipple), browner nipples and areola (especially after pregnancy), wide oval areola, small circular areola. The areola have little bumps on them. Some people develop a third or extra nipples underneath the breasts or on the stomach, which are often mistaken for moles. Some can tie their breasts in a knot behind their head. This is not recommended on public transport.

I think Denis Leary, an American comedian, speaks for most men when he says, 'I don't understand the fascination with breast implants. I like the real thing, no matter what the size. I like big ones. I like small ones. I think I even like the smaller ones better than the big ones. I love all shapes, all sizes. I love the ones that are shaped like golf balls, I love the ones that are shaped like teardrops. I like the melons and the pears, the footballs and the ferns. I love them all, as long as they're real.' Thank you, Dennis.

Lumps and bumps

You should get to know the shape and feel of your breasts, which may be naturally slightly lumpy. Then, when you examine your breasts by look and touch after each period (when they are least likely to be retaining fluid) you can notice any changes. You can develop breast cancer at any age. But it's rarer in women under 30 and more common in women as they get older, and those who have a history of it in the family.

A breast lump may be an early sign of a problem that can be cured easily or it may be nothing to worry about. But if it does develop – and size is no indication of how dangerous a lump is – it could result in incurable cancer. Early detection of breast cancer means a much higher chance of survival.

More than 25,000 new cases of breast cancer are reported in the UK every year. Many will die of it but live normal lives for another 20 or 30 years. Others will be 'cured', if they have come early for treatment. More than 15,000 women die of breast cancer each year in the UK. Others with advanced cancer can be cured but the radiation therapy can make them unable to have children afterwards.

Many women have the small lump removed rather than an entire breast. Tell all the women in your family especially those who are over 40 that they should get a free examination at a Family Planning clinic (see back of book) or their doctor. A breast examination can be done once a year by a doctor at the same time as a Pap smear, or during a visit for something else.

So if a lump appears and it's still there after a period, go and have it looked at. You won't need surgery to confirm a diagnosis. The doctor will put a fine needle into the lump and take out some fluid. It can be a pretty scary thing to go through, so take a friend or relative in with you if you like.

You might have heard that Asian women are at less risk. This is only true for women of Asian origin in their country of heritage and eating a traditional diet.

There is an opinion that breastfeeding and the caressing, manipulating and stimulation of breasts and nipples helps to guard against cancer. (Hmmmm. Wacko.) It is known that pregnancy does something to breasts to make them less likely to develop cancer, unless there is a history of it in the family. And yet the US Centre for Disease Control found that three-quarters of cases were in women with no publicised risk factors. The only real way to stop it is eternal vigilance and to get any lumps checked out immediately – weeks can be crucial.

Disturbingly, no study has ever been done about whether the

family history of shared breast cancer is due to heredity or shared environment or diet. The latest tip is a high-fibre diet may help. The jump in breast cancer in the last 20 years is often attributed partly to a higher-fat diet. Many researchers in the US now believe that may be due to the level of agricultural pesticide residue in meat and other foods. There is increasing evidence that carcinogens come from various sources such as industry, its production and toxic waste, and pesticides.

These researchers suggest – and it can't hurt – we should get rid of all the synthetic chemicals possible in our immediate and community environments, especially organochlorins such as DDT, PCBs, CFCs and dioxins. (According to the US Environmental Protection agency, counties with hazardous waste sites are 6.5 times more likely to have high breast-cancer rates than other counties. Two counties routinely saturated with aerial spraying of the pesticide DDT during the 1950s report the highest breast-cancer rates in the US.)

Despite the money spent on breast cancer, most is going on the idea of 'cures' and detection of a problem already there, the emphasis has not been on prevention. One of the best steps towards preventing cancers may be to join an environmental group that works against the dangerous use and dumping of toxic chemicals and find a book of hints for 'greener' living.

Inverted nipples One in ten women has inverted nipples. This means the nipple is in recess rather than protruding. Most women find theirs can be popped out for breastfeeding. A small safe plastic cup with a vacuum effect can be used to draw out the nipple and 'train' it to point outwards. This can also be done by gently pulling the nipple out each day. ('*Hello*

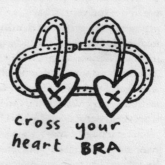

cross your heart BRA

90

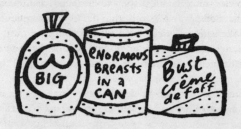

there!') Some doctors may suggest a surgical alternative but that should be a very last resort. If your nipple suddenly inverts, having never done so before, see a doctor.

Bust firming 'I must, I must improve my bust,' goes the desperate chant of women doing silly pectoral exercises that cannot 'improve' or enlarge breasts. This desperation can lead them to frighteningly expensive and totally useless creams like the thrilling Guaranteed Sabrina Cream and the New Curvy Girl Method which were flogged in *True Confessions* magazines and comics of the 1950s and 1960s.

'You'll go to gay places – be admired by men, envied by women' promised the Curvy Girl ad, which never mentioned what method you'd get for your money: an ointment, a lotion? A wish and a prayer? 'I have gained three inches in 28 days' went the testimonials for Sabrina Cream (all strangely anonymous). The rather racy-sounding Lady Godiva cream promised an eye-popping four-inch gain in 28 days along with 'admiration, popularity, and affection'.

At least five mail-order companies were offering the three-inches-in-thirty-days cream during the 1960s. One can only presume that if it worked, Sabrina, Babs O'Rourke, Paula Rae and her cohorts would still be household names. Or were they just the same person with different post-office boxes? And were they really women? Or just weaselly men in grubby offices, getting cigar ash in their bourbon and signing themselves Babs?

These days Sabrina creams have pretendy French and almost scientific names: *galbeor harmonie* (*galber* is French for 'to shape or curve'), *gel multi-tenseur buste* (breast shape and firmness), and the simply stupid 'bust modelling' and 'contouring'. This is because it's illegal to advertise something silly like 'will add three inches'.

No cream or lotion in the world will firm or shape or enlarge or reduce your breasts. In previous decades protein drinks were sold which just put on weight everywhere, including the bust. The companies claim that taut, healthy skin helps prevent sagging and that all these creams moisturise and tighten the skin. So all a 'bust firming' gel

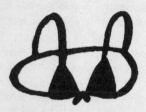

might (*might*) do is simply tighten up the *skin* very temporarily, as a mud pack or egg white would do. And they cost a lot more than mud.

The ads – regurgitated by beauty pages as 'new' information on a product – are the usual faffing on about firming plant proteins and vitamin A and hop extracts, collagen and moisturisers. One magazine, in writing about these creams under the headline 'Cultivating Curves' (a big lie), quoted the founder and president of Clarins, Jacques Coutin-Clarins, as calling the skin a 'natural bra' because of its 'vital role in shaping the bust'. This is a truly astonishing piece of stupidity. I suppose legs are nature's thigh boots and the bum is a natural pair of undies? Go and have a good lie down, Jacques.

My favourite advertised way of changing your breasts is the cassette tape called *Natural Breast Enlargement* you can buy in America. You listen to the tapes for three months to overcome your problems with maximum breast development supposedly caused by trauma during puberty (and excuse me, but who doesn't have trauma during puberty?! Which planet have *they* been sent to?).

It is expensive and tells you stuff like: 'Your breasts become whatever they're willed to be. You are the authority over your breasts. You can do it. You are a winner...You forgive yourself for not developing to your fullest. Large, full breasts make you feel satisfied,

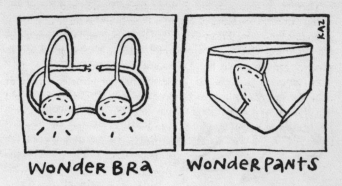

WONDER BRA   WONDER PANTS

fulfilled and vital...Your breasts grow like ripening fruit. They're warm and they're growing...there is a permanent tightness and firmness.' And may I just add, 'Liar, liar, their pants are on fire'?

Bras In the 1920s bras flattened out the breasts. In the 1950s they had padded bras called 'falsies' or stuffed hankies down there. Now we have 'dream bras' and 'wonder bras' instead, which are really just...well, falsies: up to £30 a bra. The wonder bra (what next, wonder pants with false bulges for men?) has most of the padding underneath the breast, pushing it up into an unnatural cleavage.

The media plays along. 'Headlines declaring "The bust is back" have sent lingerie companies into manufacturing overdrive as they respond to the growing demand from customers for underwear that looks

> I hate my breasts as they are very big and very uncomfortable. Difficult to buy clothes. But girls are always complaining about not having enough. I'd prefer small ones any day.
>
> Lois, 22

anything but beige,' blatted one newspaper fashion page. But that's the wrong way round. The lingerie manufacturers buy advertising space, send out glossy pictures, put out press releases and advertise and *hence* the headlines 'The bust is back' (where did it go?). And *Vogue* magazine has been even worse. 'Small breasts are back: making the most of them,' its front cover shrieked in 1993, sending us all scurry-

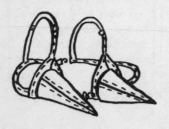

ing to the cutlery drawer to see if our old small breasts were there waiting to be taken for a spin.

Vogue went on about how to 'improve the look of the *décolletage*' (the area between the breasts) by exfoliation. 'Unfortunately, there are few advised surgical treatments to correct this highly vulnerable area of the body.' What a vile notion. Dermabrasion and chemical peels were described as an option, despite a warning by dermatologists that the area is the most prone to scarring on the entire body.

'Well, thank God for make-up,' prattles a witless *Vogue*. 'Some brown shading between the breasts to add the effect of cleavage and a veil of powder such as Clinique's Superpowder all over the *décolletage* and neck' (just don't shake your boosies near any kryptonite). *Vogue*'s article on *décolletage* mentioned no fewer than 12 specific cosmetic products recommended for the breast area.

Sales of one particular padded bra, with the pads underneath to push up the breasts, were said to be (like the breasts) alarmingly high. One journalist gushed (or regurgitated), 'The secret of the [bra] which ensures maximum uplift and a perfect shape in plunging necklines, is attributed to its 42 components, compared with only 21 in conventional bras.' No, it isn't. It's attributed to the fact that it's got a whacking great bit of false padding in it. And who decides what is a perfect shape, anyway?

> My breasts are too pointy.
>
> Lindy, 15

Sports bras are a good idea, especially to avoid annoying bouncing, sore breasts, and tearing or stretching of tissue. The good ones, made from cotton, will temporarily flatten out the breasts and have a T-shaped or crossover back, echoing the 1920s bras.

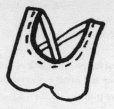

Some women feel the need to wear a bra only before their period, others never. Wearing a bra will not stop breasts becoming less youthful as you get older. One surgeon found that 60 of his patients stopped having chronic neck and chest pain when they stopped wearing their bras. These women had too much pressure on their bra straps and nearly half of them decided they wouldn't bother with bras any more.

Big ones These are physically uncomfortable for many girls, who find that large breasts disadvantage them so they face prejudice based on appearance and ignorance similar to racism.

Many girls and women with large breasts find they are rarely looked in the face by new acquaintances. 'Hey, my face is up here,' some of them say. Sometimes the teasing at school is agonising. The best revenge a large-breasted girl can have is not to give in to any stereotypes and to be proudly herself. Friends should be enlisted against the idiots wherever possible. (More hints in the Body Police section.) Large breasts which cause back problems can be reduced with surgery. Patients should find out from their doctor whether they will lose any nipple sensation or the ability to breastfeed after the operation.

Comedian Anita Wise says, 'A lot of guys think the larger a woman's breasts are, the less intelligent she is...I think the larger the woman's breasts are, the less intelligent the men become.'

> As I am continuously reminded, I have my grandmother's shape, short, broad hips and shoulders and a thicker waist than some. Where the big bust came from the family records don't tell me. At school I was constantly teased; at least every day someone would make a comment. It got to the point I couldn't look at myself without feeling sick. Guys were a problem too, chasing me for all the wrong reasons. It's nice to be kissed at the movies instead of groped.
>
> Jade, 19

95

Further information

Breast Cancer Care will send you free information about breast self-examination, lumps and cancer. *See list at end of book also.*

If you have been diagnosed with cancer find a support group and seek advice from women who have been through it.

Greenpeace and Friends of the Earth all work against pesticides and toxic chemicals in our environment. They are in the phone book.

Do I have normal thighs?

Are your thighs ruining your love life? So, you last had a date when bubble skirts were in fashion and your most recent human contact was an old age pensioner falling on you in the bus? Could your thighs be to blame?

Could it be that Mr Right passed you in the street only yesterday and was about to sweep you off your feet, shower you with rose petals and canter about on a big white horse until you considered calling the RSPCA, but just as he was on the point of handing over his heart and his credit cards and insist that he couldn't go on without you, he noticed that you had thin, taut thighs?

'Dang,' muttered Mr Right as he strode away, his ripply bits, well, rippling and the cashmere overcoat you could have borrowed swirling around him in a tragic way. 'If only that woman had thighs like the girlies in the Rubens paintings, I would have been her slave for the rest of my life, and always left the toilet seat down and everything.'

Well I'm sorry, but it's far-fetched. When a man is feeling frisky he does not think to himself: 'Good Lord! That woman's thighs do not look like the legs of a 12-year-old fashion model! I shall vow never to love her physically!'

No, by the stage of things when a man is feeling your thighs, he is more likely to have disengaged the thinking part of his brain entirely, which is why you might like to have a condom handy. The warm, soft skin on the inside of a woman's thigh – whether plump or thin – is liable to be driving him wild with desire. Honest.

If, at this point, you are thinking to yourself, 'Oh my God, he's thinking that my thighs aren't perfect so I'll just tense them up to feign a bit of muscle tone,' you will not be entering into the spirit of this crazed lust thing. And I'm sorry, but crazed lust beats jogging almost any way you look at it.

Worrying about being well groomed and svelte in the middle of sex (or if you don't have sex, substitute being at the pool or beach with friends) is not conducive to having a good time. It is difficult to achieve orgasm or perfect the butterfly stroke while trying to repair one's mascara and blending three lipsticks for shading purposes. (Well, I *hear* it's difficult.)

Some women have become expert at drawing attention away from their thighs. Dangling from the chandelier clad only in a dab of whipped cream and shouting, 'Come over here, big boy!' is popular. So is shouting, 'Look! Over there! A violent football match!' when removing the lower half of one's clothes.

Which only goes to prove that if you are one of these tortured souls, it is not your thighs ruining your love life but your self-esteem problem. So we're just going to get this out in the open, *right now*.

Big thighs are okay Anybody who tries to convince you otherwise probably stands to gain, usually financially, from making you feel hideous about your legs. If you like your thighs the way they are, or accept them as just another part of you, you're not going to spend money in trying to change them, disguise them, read about them or buy new clothes that are supposed to make you look like a trained whippet.

The people telling you you'd look better with thinner thighs are not going to ask you out, watch a video with you, be coerced into giving you a foot massage, take you home when you're not feeling well or laugh at your jokes. No, they just want to sell you massage treatments, breakfast cereal, weight-loss programs, laxatives, frozen 'diet' meals, gym mem-

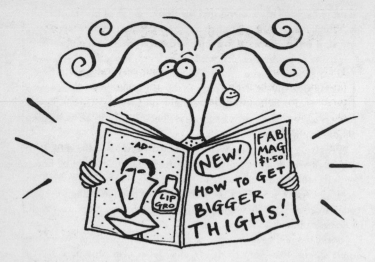

bership, magazines and useless lotions and potions. They don't even want to meet you.

It is precisely because thin thighs are not the average state of womanhood that they are held up as the ideal. If most of us had perfectly fine, thin thighs instead of perfectly fine, rounded thighs, they'd be calling us scrawny and trying to convince us to buy some products which would bulk up our legs. Which they – the advertisers – will do, if they think there's money in it.

> I am always six kilos overweight. Call me thunderthighs. You could say I go through life constantly looking for ways to improve myself and I'm almost convinced that without my dimply thighs and droopy bottom, I wouldn't need those damn [magazine] articles.
>
> Marie, 24

What about those models? Hey, it's their *job* to have thin thighs. They are *paid* to have thin thighs. They are naturally thinner, and then they diet and exercise for hours every day to fit into their job description and those tiny frocks.

Now, let's try this short quiz to see how we're getting on:

The thigh quiz

1. My thighs are
(a) Those bits between my torso and my gorgeous little old kneesies
(b) Like magnets to a lover's soul
(c) A hazard to shipping

2. The world is a better place for the lasting contribution made to it by
(a) Aretha Franklin
(b) The Dalai Lama
(c) Elle Macpherson

3. You would rather spend four hours
(a) With a tireless lover and a bottle of champagne
(b) Seeing how many after-dinner mints you can eat in a row without throwing up
(c) Doing a mindless, repetitive exercise to tone your thighs

4. Cellulite is
(a) French for marketing opportunity
(b) Not a recognised medical condition
(c) Taking over your entire body

5. Your best feature is
(a) Your sparkling wit
(b) Your ability to throw your voice while drinking a mug of Horlicks
(c) The way you can spend an entire relationship backing out of rooms so he can't see the back of your legs

6. Of the following, one is most likely to ruin your love life
(a) Your partner has this thing for short women in chicken suits
(b) Your partner is having an affair with at least three people and all the major gender groups are covered
(c) Your thighs

7. You want to move in together but your lover hasn't seen
(a) The point
(b) *Thelma and Louise*
(c) Your legs

8. If you answered (c) to any of these questions you need
(a) A good lie down
(b) A very cunning swimsuit indeed
(c) Counselling

Top five signs that you need to get over your thigh obsession

1. It's the third date and you're still wearing the army blanket.
2. Everyone else is swimming but you're lying on a pontoon with your thighs swathed in cling wrap.
3. You think thighs should not wobble.
4. Liposuction doesn't sound utterly insane to you.
5. He says, 'You seem to be consumed with heavy sighs tonight, my love' and you think he said, 'I'm leaving you, podgy-legs'.

Who says you've got fat thighs and why?

Thighs are a major concern of women. The fearful obsession that 'my thighs are too fat' is used to sell magazines. One magazine carried the cover line 'Who's got the best and worst thighs in Hollywood?'. Inside, photographs of celebrities accompanied an article by comedian Rita Rudner called 'Hollywood thighs' which wasn't about thighs at all but about the relentless obsession with exercise in Los Angeles.

With it the magazine ran photos of women with 'truly great thighs' and 'thunderthighs', none of whom were mentioned in Ms Rudner's article. 'Great' thigh owners included Madonna, who exercises for up to five hours a day, and models Naomi Campbell and Cindy Crawford, who are built thin and also exercise more than any sensible person would have time for.

The 'thunderthighs' owners included Paula Abdul (a dancer!), Whitney Houston (who I'm pretty sure was photographed at a time not unadjacent to a pregnancy) and the Duchess of York, who does not, to my knowledge, live in Los Angeles, but her skirt blew up

— What exercises can I do at home to get rid of cellulite around my bum?
— Why bother? It's female. Accept yourself. Celebrate yourself – that's what's beautiful!

Graffiti in University Union building

when a photographer was around. This is pure bitchiness, which is presumably supposed to make readers with normal, curvy thighs feel good that celebrities have similar ones. But it's all under the big banner of 'thunderthighs': hardly a soothing definition of perfectly normal legs.

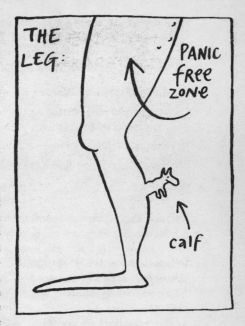

The next issue of the magazine had a cover line proclaiming that some men love 'fat thighs'. In the article the man who wrote it did not call thighs 'fat' at all. He didn't even think they were. Was this the magazine's definition: if not thin, then it must be fat? I asked an editor at the magazine why the word 'fat' was used on the cover but not inside. She looked at me as if I were supremely stupid. 'Because it sells magazines,' she said. Women who think they have fat thighs will buy the magazine to read about which men like 'fat' thighs but their thighs are still defined as 'fat' when they are perfectly normal. (There is a definite definition problem here.)

I hate my thighs.

Anonymous

Because of roller skating I have big muscly legs and I used to hate that about my legs because it made the top of them look fat, but I have found out guys actually like that.

Romany, 18

But perhaps things are improving. Previously, a magazine had trumpeted in a cover line that it had photos of the supermodels 'who used to be fat'.

Of course, they didn't use to be 'fat' at all, as the article pointed out. They had simply lost more weight from their already underweight frames. When taken to task by a reader's letter for this ('How can we accept the way we are, reading magazine articles like these?') the magazine apologised, pleading irony.

'We're sorry!' the editor wrote on the letters page. 'You misunderstood our use of the word fat. Our point was that these models could never and should never have been considered fat, yet with this trend towards "super-waifs", even already slim models are starving themselves into super-skinniness.'

> Well the bits I don't like about myself would be my thighs but that comes with being a female.
>
> Karen, 14

In the same issue, the magazine gave valuable space to publicising a call to women to write to me if they wanted to contribute to this book about body image.

So the magazines are trying to help within the bounds of what they know will boost sales and keep their advertisers happy. Magazines will not change cover lines, including the word 'fat', when they know it will sell more copies.

But magazines are not vehicles of social change, they are commercial ventures. We cannot wait for magazines to independently show a lead when it is not rewarded by sales. But we can read them more selectively

> A whole group of us girls walked into maths class and the guys kept saying 'thunderthighs' to one of my friends. This destroyed all her self-confidence and she told me that she cries herself to sleep every night.
>
> Daisy, 14

and more critically. Read the magazines you like but don't take everything they say as gospel. When you see the word 'fat' on the cover of a magazine, it's not necessarily accurate or relevant to your body – it's a sales tool. You do not have to accept that definition of your thighs or of yourself.

The great cellulite scam Cellulite is the name given to the dimply-looking fat deposits found on the thighs or legs of almost all women. It's not a name recognised by the medical profession, but it's sure as hell a 'condition', 'affliction' or 'problem' according to the

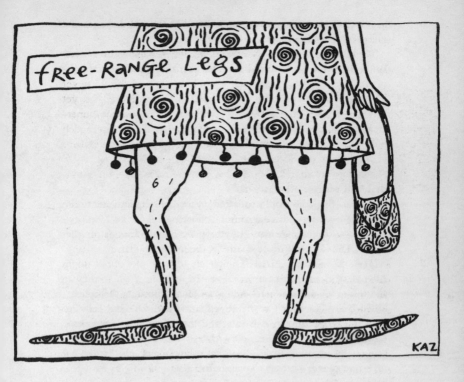

cosmetics industry. On the latest available figures, American women spend $170 million a year on cellulite creams, lotions and 'treatments'.

Most of the information about cellulite comes from the US. An American professor of Internal Medicine says, 'If you're prone to getting it, cellulite will show up no matter how hard you exercise.' A New York plastic surgeon says cellulite is hereditary and more common in women who have dramatic weight reductions.

A spokesperson for the US Food and Drugs Administration says some creams can reduce the signs of cellulite or improve the appearance by temporarily tightening the skin. You would get the exact same effect with glue or egg white. The difference made by the creams is barely visible, or invisible, but the skin feels tighter.

Perhaps the most damning news comes from a clinical assistant professor at an American medical school who exposed the fraud of expensive rubbing devices, mitts and creams.

Stimulating the skin by scrubbing, he says, will increase the circulation and make the skin look smoother because it is causing the skin to swell up. All that happens is *low-level bruising and swelling*.

'People who fall for these creams misunderstand the structure of their bodies,' says another New York plastic surgeon. 'There's no cream in the world that will restore elasticity to your skin.' She adds that lotions and creams cannot eliminate toxins, break up body fat or have a diuretic effect.

> Don't think that thin people don't have cellulite – we do!
>
> Catherine, 17

Let's get something clear. *All* grown-up women have fat on their thighs. This does not make them 'fat thighs', or too fat.

Marie Claire magazine has completely lost the plot about thighs. After all, the cellulite scam was invented in France, where they are allowed to sell a cream marketed as a Quick Slimming Complexe – called Body Contour Cream elsewhere – with fat- and cellulite-reducing properties. In Australia and the US such a 'fat-melting' claim would have to be proved with tests and studies, so the advertising in those countries does not make the same claims. *Marie Claire* magazine awarded it Best Cream of the Year in a vote by European beauty editors.

Another *Marie Claire* article about cellulite epitomises the very worst of 'beauty reporting'. Its report read: 'Between the ages of fifteen and 50, up to 80 per cent of women are susceptible to cellulite, according to shape specialists Elancyl.'

Shape specialists? What's a shape specialist? In this case it's a cosmetics company that makes a fortune out of selling cellulite 'treatments'. Shape specialists, if you don't mind me saying, my arse.

Cellulite tends to accumulate, says the company, before menopause, in contraceptive pill users, during pregnancy, in times of stress, during emotional trauma, in smokers, and in people who don't exercise a lot. It makes perfect sense if you recognise that cellulite is really normal deposits of padding that all women – even thin women – have (menopause, smoking and stress aside).

Another magazine listed 'treatments' including lying in sand for 30 minutes at a time, saunas, a friction rub (well we know what *that* does), marine algae wraps, aromatherapy, reflexology, an entire body exfoliation, diet, exercise, not getting tense, electrodes attached to 'the parts of the body needing treatment' to stimulate muscles instead of exercising (eek!), vibration machines, herbal oils, being attached to a thermal heat machine, aerobics, step aerobics, weightlifting, and lotions (naming all the cosmetics companies' major products) with ingredients including 'liposomes', 'non-ionic microspheres', 'marine life derivatives', 'kaolin' (which is ordinary clay), 'centella asiatica', 'micro-reservoirs of collagen', unspecified 'key ingredients' and sunflower oil.

Then the magazine listed seven separate thigh moisturisers all by cosmetic company and trade name. Just another ad.

'It may be worth investing in Shiseido's Body Exfoliating Scrub [£20] too. Active plant extracts such as the circulatory aid butcher's broom, as well as ivy and caffeine (which both have contouring properties) are common anti-cellulite ingredients; sometimes they are combined with synthetic chemicals to make their fat-busting powers more potent', the magazine continued shamelessly. Oo-er.

Let's just examine that statement like the new detectives we are. Will we be bamboozled by the pseudo science? What's an active plant extract anyway – something from a potplant that goes jogging? It's just jargon.

And the circulatory aids – well, anything is a circulatory aid if you're vigorously rubbing it in and scrubbing – do that anywhere on your skin without a product and you'll get an improvement in circulation as blood rushes to the surface. In fact, German lederhosen dances in which you slap your thighs will probably have the same effect, although you'd have to listen to polka music.

And as for the phrase 'fat-busting', it sounds like an ad, is hardly scientific and is not backed up by any evidence. In fact, it is a slogan and nothing more.

We have been conned. The multi-million dollar cosmetics companies, aided by women's magazines who have swallowed their propaganda hook, line and sinker, are trying to convince us our natural curves and padding are 'unsightly'.

My friend Stephanie was told at a Clarins counter that there was 'nothing worse than cellulite'. 'How about nuclear war?' she replied. The saleswoman looked sceptical.

Stretch marks When an area of the body gets bigger or smaller quickly – like when you develop bigger hips, breasts and thighs at puberty – it often leaves stretch marks.

This also happens with rapid weight gain and loss, so it's common among dieters. And lots of pregnant women get stretch marks on their tummy, bottom, and legs as everything gets bigger in readiness for the baby.

> I have so many stretch marks.
>
> Sally-Anne, 17

Like 'cellulite' and body shape, a tendency to stretch marks is hereditary. This is not an excuse to go and shout at your parents. As if you need one.

Some doctors and herbalists say that people deficient in zinc and vitamin B6 are more prone to the marks, and vitamin-E tablets and creams are recommended by women who have used them during pregnancy. But other dermatologists say that there is usually only a tiny amount of vitamin E in a lotion and it's not certain it can penetrate the skin.

The marks are often in the form of red or purple lines, but over time, they will fade to a shimmer and become hardly noticeable unless you're inspecting yourself closely with a magnifying glass or fretting about it.

> I have stretch marks on my hips, thighs, and bum. I hate them but I am slowly getting used to them 'cos they are fading.
>
> Maeve, 15

By the time we're all grown up, almost all women have them, many without ever noticing. Others hide, wearing shorts and refusing to go swimming and missing out on a feeling of freedom and fun.

Do I have normal periods?

Visit from a friend To understand periods, you need to understand that a woman's life is like a cycle (although not very much like a unicycle) and that after puberty, usually in our early teens, we start having a monthly menstrual cycle. This goes on until menopause in middle age.

Every month the body makes an egg, which if fertilised by sperm will become an embryo – the start of a baby. (We can stop this from happening by not losing our minds with lust without using some form of contraception.)

Menstruating, or a period, or Fred, or being 'on the rag' is what happens when the body realises you haven't fertilised the nice egg it made for you and the egg and the extra thickening on the inside of your womb – where an embryo would have grown – is expelled through 'bleeding'.

The amount of the average bleed is only 50 millilitres over two to seven days, although it often seems to be more. Periods can start from the age of 10 to 17-ish and visit regularly until you're between 45 and 55. All these statistics vary widely from woman to woman and there is a wide variation of 'normal'.

Anything which changes radically for the woman may be abnormal for her like suddenly getting heavy periods, or a shorter cycle each time. A change for just one cycle can usually be ignored.

If you haven't ovulated (made the egg) you can still get a period. Some people miss a few periods here and there, others get one every 28 days regular as anything, and some people have one every three months or three weeks: all these can be 'normal'.

Many religions and cultures held or even still hold that menstruation is a taboo. Women are banned from churches and kitchens during their period. This is because people who don't fully understand the process think it is unclean and bizarre. Given that it will happen to more than half the population during most of their lives, this kind of attitude is pretty pathetic.

The embarrassment extends to coy advertising. Some of you may be wondering why they advertise pads and tampons by putting blue ink on them. So are the rest of us. The only person who ever had a blue period was Picasso. Don't be embarrassed about your period. (Unless it's blue.)

Here are some things you can do SIMULTANEOUSLY with having your period (but only if you really want to): have sex, swim, have showers or baths, drive a large passenger train and dance. Although I wouldn't recommend trying to drive a passenger train and dance simultaneously. (I be that party pooper.)

This is not to say that when your period first happens it isn't amazing and special and kind of scary, even if you've been warned about

PAD WITH WINGS

Your Menstrual Calendar

Keep track of the little euphemism through the year. Easy to find out how regular you are, or if your period is late. Circle each day of your period throughout the year and watch your pattern emerge. This chart should not be used for contraception unless you want to have vast quantities of babies. If you need contraception, use condoms instead.

Jan 1	29	26	25	21	18	15	13	9	5	3	31	27	25
2	30	27	26	22	19	16	14	10	6	4		28	26
3	31	28	27	23	20	17	15	11	7	5	Nov 1	29	27
4	Feb 1		28	24	21	18	16	12	8	6	2	30	28
5	2	Mar 1	29	25	22	19	17	13	9	7	3	Dec 1	29
6	3	2	30	26	23	20	18	14	10	8	4	2	30
7	4	3	31	27	24	21	19	15	11	9	5	3	31
8	5	4		28	25	22	20	16	12	10	6	4	Jan 1
9	6	5	Apr 1	29	26	23	21	17	13	11	7	5	2
10	7	6	2	30	27	24	22	18	14	12	8	6	3
11	8	7	3		28	25	23	19	15	13	9	7	4
12	9	8	4	May 1	29	26	24	20	16	14	10	8	5
13	10	9	5	2	30	27	25	21	17	15	11	9	6
14	11	10	6	3	31	28	26	22	18	16	12	10	7
15	12	11	7	4	Jun 1	29	27	23	19	17	13	11	8
16	13	12	8	5	2	30	28	24	20	18	14	12	9
17	14	13	9	6	3	Jul 1	29	25	21	19	15	13	10
18	15	14	10	7	4	2	30	26	22	20	16	14	11
19	16	15	11	8	5	3	31	27	23	21	17	15	12
20	17	16	12	9	6	4		28	24	22	18	16	13
21	18	17	13	10	7	5	Aug 1	29	25	23	19	17	14
22	19	18	14	11	8	6	2	30	26	24	20	18	15
23	20	19	15	12	9	7	3	31	27	25	21	19	16
24	21	20	16	13	10	8	4		28	26	22	20	17
25	22	21	17	14	11	9	5	Sep 1	29	27	23	21	18
26	23	22	18	15	12	10	6	2	30	28	24	22	19
27	24	23	19	16	13	11	7	3	Oct 1	29	25	23	20
28	25	24	20	17	14	12	8	4	2	30	26	24	21

This menstrual calendar is in lines of 28 days, the 'average' time between periods. But some modern girls get a period every 16 days or every couple of months.

it. It's part of becoming a woman. And yes, it is natural that you can smell the blood after it has contact with the air. It is very unlikely that anyone else can, although dogs, with their incredibly acute, inhuman sense of smell, will often try and put their noses in your crotch at that time of the month. Which is one reason why you should only cultivate friendships with people who have short dogs.

Menstrual diary Because your period is an indication of whether or not you are pregnant, as well as general health, and sometimes a mood predictor, it's a good idea to keep a record of it. Include details and dates of any changes in the colour (what kind of red or brown), amount or consistency of the blood, any pre-menstrual symptoms, the nature and times of any pain and, once you've established a pattern, when the next period is likely.

This can be very helpful to you and your doctor – and those close to you who can make plans to go interstate whenever you're premenstrual. My *Modern Girl's Diary* produced in Australia each year has a menstrual diary at the back. But I suppose I can't flog one to everybody in the world, so here's another one you can cut out or photocopy and keep somewhere you'll use it.

Don't be surprised if you find that your period ends up synchronised with the other women you live, work or study with. Nobody is quite sure why this happens, although they suspect some sort of unconscious armpit sniffing. Personally, I think it's a kind of subconscious etiquette. 'Let's get this PMT stuff over and done with all at once. Behold the bite marks on the furniture! Express an opinion if ye dare! Cower in terror, ye visitors to the house of HELL!'

Pre-menstrual tension or syndrome (PMT or PMS) Pre-menstrual symptoms include fluid retention that results in bigger, tighter and sorer breasts, bloated stomach, low self-esteem, increased weight everywhere, pimples usually before, but sometimes also during and/or after the period, moodiness, clumsiness, back pain, leg pain, being furious, loss of concentration abilities, depression, a bizarrely determined need for chocolate, confusion and general

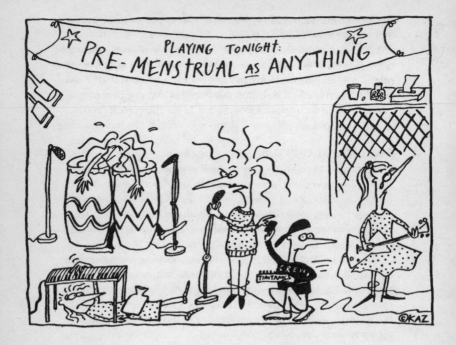

unspecific crabbiness and tears. Also insomnia, headaches, and more rarely, manic behaviour like cleaning out the inside of the fridge even though it isn't your turn.

This is to do with the complex relationship between the mysterious HORMONES, oestrogen and progesterone. More research into the syndrome (or syndromes) is needed. Some doctors still will not acknowledge its existence because it is so hard to measure. Studies have shown that women are more likely to commit crimes or attempt suicide just before their period, not to mention more likely to eat a block of chocolate approximately the size of Shropshire.

One idea is to flag your pre-menstrual days to your family or housemates by hanging a red scarf or flag (or bedspread if things are really tough) on the calendar or on the fridge for the duration. Then when they say, 'Good morning!' and you bark, 'Start that kind of talk with me and I'll run you through with a bayonet!' they can just ignore you instead of calling the police. On the other hand, maybe they should have called the police.

Take your menstrual diary to a doctor or naturopath who can help you decide what is best for your symptoms. You may have to rifle the neighbourhood for the right 'health professional' – ask around. Naturopaths and doctors often suggest evening primrose oil capsules, along with vitamin B6 in doses larger than usually recommended. Both these things are cheaper in bulk at the supermarket than at health food shops. Naturopaths are likely to ask you many questions, aiming to prescribe treatments best suited to your individual needs. The times to take tablets (just during pre-menstrual time or all month) will vary between women.

Diuretics, which make you wee a lot and lose the fluid retention, may also be prescribed. Chemical ones can strip the body of potassium and magnesium, and herbal ones such as celery juice or celery and juniper herbal tablets may work less dramatically. Because unripe juniper berries may cause kidney problems, you should follow the packet instructions and not use the tablets continuously for more than two months. They should not be used by people with kidney disease. Dandelion leaf tea is good and contains plenty of potassium and magnesium. (Personally I think it tastes like boiled grass clippings.) Beware of taking too many diuretics, which will dehydrate your body.

Also, not being stressed can help as the uterus spasms will not be so painful. Stress can alter the state of our hormones and bring on an imbalance. This is why some people swear by yoga, massage, exercise and other relaxation methods.

Other medications include anti–inflammatory drugs, chamomile, raspberry leaf, peppermint, fresh ginger and red clover teas, acupuncture, calcium tablets, aspirin, essential fatty acids other than primrose oil, minerals, and progesterone therapy.

PMT sufferers should eat between meals! And have little snacks often in the days before their period. Eating fruit, raw veggies, nuts or soya milk will keep up protein and cut excessive, yo-yoing blood-sugar levels. This will stave off the chocolate cravings, too. Cut down on salt which aids fluid retention, caffeine which will make you wired, and sugar which can spiral you into more sugar cravings. Tobacco and alcohol just confuse the situation (as is their wont).

It never arrived There are several reasons for not getting your period including pregnancy, breastfeeding, ill-health perhaps due to drugs, severe physical or psychological stress, over-exercise and poor nutrition. If you have not started having periods by the age of 17 see a doctor or go to a family-planning clinic. But don't panic and remember, everyone is different. If you miss two periods in your usual cycle, it should be checked out.

Period pain This is really common. 'Cramps' are simply that – often just before or on the first day of the period spasms of the uterus help expel the blood.

The trick is not to put up with very bad pain, or mask it with very strong painkillers or anti-spasm drugs. It is your body telling you there is something wrong and not 'a woman's lot' that must be endured. Do not put up with pain which interferes with your lifestyle and cannot be controlled by recommended doses of low-level painkillers. This pain may include vomiting, nausea, aching or stabbing pains before, during and after a period, violent cramps or similarly awful pains at ovulation.

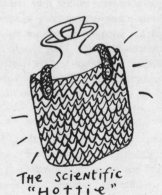

The scientific "Hottie"

Find a sympathetic doctor and/or naturopath and make them earn your money. If your doctor tells you the pain is normal or neurotic behaviour, or something that women must put up with, lurch across the desk with your eyes rolling and attempt to strangle him or her, screaming politely, 'Is this NORMAL?!'

Trust your instincts and insist on a referral to a menstruation specialist. You may be easily relieved of your pain by a course of tablets, or find that you have a treatable menstrual disorder such as endometriosis, in which some blood leaks back through the Fallopian tubes instead of out of the body. Or pelvic inflammatory disease, in

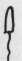

which the tubes become damaged and eventually blocked. If PID or endometriosis are not treated they may cause terrible pain and infertility later on.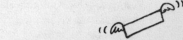

 As for your 'average' cramps – herbal remedies, heat (such as a hot-water bottle, known by its scientific name, the 'hottie'), swimming and yoga exercises have helped some women to banish period pain.

Tampons and Towels Always use the lowest absorbency for your needs and try to use towels whenever possible to reduce the risk of Toxic Shock Syndrome, associated with tampons, which can be fatal. Towels also allow a more natural flow. Tampons can absorb natural moisture as well as blood in the vagina, so at least use towels at night during your period. If your tampon is hard to remove, there's not enough fluid to make it necessary, so swap to a light towel. Tampons should not be left in for more than six hours and never overnight.

Using tampons for the first time will not mean that you are no longer a virgin. Don't force anything that hurts. Follow the instructions in the packet and don't be shy of gently stretching your vagina, over time, with your (clean) fingers. (Lock the door first!)

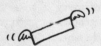

Further reading

The best book about what happens to your body is *The New Our Bodies Ourselves,* by Angela Phillips and Jill Rakusen (2nd British edition, first published by Penguin Books, 1989).

Women's and community health centres should have specific pamphlets on menstruation.

Do I have normal skin?

Acne and pimples Experts disagree about exactly what causes all pimples. (It makes you wonder why we bother having experts,
really.) Hormones definitely play the major part, which is why you
might get pimples before your period. Almost all experts now say
eating four blocks of chocolate has nothing to do with pimples. Only
a handful still say that food is a factor but we have locked them all in
the broom cupboard.

You can probably work out whether food, stress, smoking and
hormone cycles and irregularities affect your skin by keeping track of
them and any subsequent mad, blind pimple fest your skin responds
with.

You can keep pimples down to a dull roar by washing carefully
with soap and water as often as you need, to cut down the oiliness in
your skin. I know everybody says it, but don't touch pimples because
it can cause infection which may result in scarring. Get out of the
habit of resting your chin in the palm of your hand, for example.
Try not to squeeze pimples, especially if they're not ready, because
this can leave bruising and even scars.

Acne creams from the chemist
can abrade the skin, making it
peel away. Be careful you don't
use too much. Very hard drying
agents such as alcohol and per-
oxide can also cause nasty-look-
ing skin peeling around a pimple.

The major problem, feral
hormones, is very common
during adolescence and not
unknown thereafter. At puberty, hormones enlarge the glands
and get them to produce more
oil. This can continue throughout your life, particularly before

> I used to get called names like 'space face
> crater', 'Pizza Hut', 'spotty' and more. This
> made me feel extremely sad, distressed and
> very hurt. I kept myself as healthy as possi-
> ble and did the right things but my skin is
> still rough and has open pores. People say
> I'm pretty anyway. I feel awful, though.
> When I look at the models in magazines I
> feel cheated.
>
> **Anonymous**

a period, or while on the contraceptive pill. A hormone imbalance
can be helped by a doctor or naturopath.

Some natural therapists believe that toxins such as smoke, alcohol, many drugs including prescribed and illegal, anaesthetic and environmental poisoning may cause pimples as the body tries every way it can to get rid of them. Most dermatologists disagree.

All dermatologists *do* agree that despite the rumour, drinking more water will have *no effect* on your skin.

Eighty per cent of people get pimples and there's a plan to send the rest to another planet as soon as we have the technology. For most people, the pimple stage passes. If you are concerned, you can get a referral to a dermatologist from your local doctor. Make sure that any drug treatment is fully explained to you, including risks and side effects.

Steer clear of chemical skin peels. That's your top layers of skin they're ripping off your face. Peels should be done only by a qualified dermatologist – if you're really determined to submit yourself to it.

By the way, you can squeeze blackheads, but no known product has been invented that will change the size of your pores and stop them filling up again. Everybody has blackheads.

Tanning Do you want the bad news first or the good news first? We might as well get right in amongst it: skin cancer. It can kill you if it can kill 500 people a year in the UK, at last count. More than 30,000 people in the UK develop skin cancer every year. This means any mole or lump or warty thing on your body should be checked and then rechecked by a doctor if you see any changes in feel or appearance. Some skin marks are harmless and very common, such as freckles, skin tags, moles and beauty marks and spots. Melanomas – the most nasty skin cancers – usually start as flat, coloured spots. The colour may begin as, or develop to, white, red, pink, light brown, dark brown or black.

Most sun experts agree that the more sunburns you have had the more likely you are to get skin cancer.

The Imperial Cancer Research Fund and the Health Education Authority recommend staying out of the sun between 10 am and 2 pm. They'd like you to have a broad-brimmed hat that casts a solid shade all around (not a baseball cap), use a sunscreen not less than Factor 15, applied at least 15 minutes before you are in the sun, and every two hours (more if you've been in the water), hang out in the

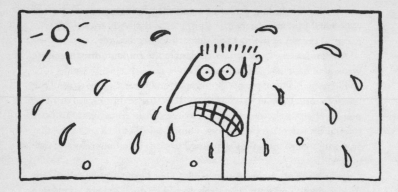

shade where possible, and wear sunglasses to British Standard 2724: 1987 so your eyeballs don't get roasted (or something to do with ultraviolet ray damage).

The biggest danger period is the middle of the day at any time and especially from June to September, when UV (ultraviolet) radiation is stronger than it is the rest of the year. But don't forget that surfaces like concrete and snow can throw up massive UV reflections and burn you.

When applying sunscreen, don't forget your fiddly bits such as lips, ears, backs of the knees, toes, elbows and the back of your neck. The upper back, which is difficult to reach by yourself, is a common place for melanoma skin cancers.

Fake tans Who was that giant carrot? That was me in a fake tan. The sales of fake tanning creams have risen with the awareness of the dangers of real tans. No models will tan. All of them use fake ones if required for a job.

Fake tans are scary for many reasons. One, we don't know their long-term effects. Two, they're expensive and they only last a few days. Some wash off in water. Three, they induce a false sense of security but offer no protection against real sunburn. Four, they continue the idea that a tan is fashionable, which keeps idiots out there every summer frying themselves silly. Five, they can stain clothes and furniture and six, they can make you look like a giant carrot with brown palms.

Spooky time: solariums are where fake tans are produced by sun lamps and sun beds. The Cancer Councils are rabidly opposed to them and here's why. Most solariums claim their fluorescent tubes emit only UVA (ultraviolet radiation) rays but many also emit UVB rays. Until recently it was thought that UVA rays were harmless but now we know they cause premature wrinkling. Some evidence also links them with skin cancers.

UVB rays are the most likely to cause sunburn and skin damage leading to skin cancer. UVB rays are dangerous to the eyes. Some drugs and cosmetics can increase a person's vulnerability to ultraviolet rays, including the contraceptive pill, antibiotics and tranquillizers. To remember which is which, think of it this way: UVB for burn and UVA for ageing.

Many people think they look healthier with a tan, hence the fake trend, which will be encouraged and perpetuated by images of tanned models in fashion magazines that take much of their revenue from the cosmetic companies selling fake tans. Many magazine stories have heartily recommended – even insisted on – fake tans, which their manufacturers would rather call (inaccurately) self-tans.

Bleaching Dangerous lightening and bleaching creams are available all over the world and are common and popular in European, American, Asian, African, Caribbean and other countries where people with darker skin are discriminated against, and where an Anglo-Saxon ideal of beauty and wealth is advertised or glorified. Bleaching and lightening chemicals can cause burns, premature ageing and patchy, mottled effects. And anyway, Indian, Asian, Aboriginal, African and Islander skins are beautiful just the way they are.

Do I have normal smells?

Sweating Everybody sweats. As a matter of fact, most of us sweat about one-and-a-half litres of sweat each 24 hours, without exercise. With exercise we become dripping soggy things, losing up to a litre an hour.

This is because we each have about three million sweat glands all over the body. (What was that noise? That was my mind boggling.) Tight clothes and most unnatural fabrics don't allow the sweat to evaporate, which makes for a stickier feeling.

Armpits Deodorants and anti-perspirants each work in different ways. Anti-perspirants are made from aluminium. This shrinks pores and reduces the amount of sweat able to escape from the body. Anti-perspirants are more likely to cause allergies and irritations than deodorants, which kill bacteria, the element in sweat which causes it to smell. Deodorants do not interfere with the natural process of sweating.

A natural deodorising crystal has been developed which has no chemicals or perfumes and can be rubbed under your armpits for up to a year or more. (Not that you should stand there for more than a year rubbing your armpits. Well, not unless you haven't anything else to do.)

Some people don't use deodorant or anti-perspirant at all, preferring to wash regularly. Because we all sweat differently, some people who use deodorant products may sweat more than somebody with *au naturel* pits.

Body odour from the armpits and genital areas is normal. The body produces chemical attractants from these areas to arouse sexual partners. While some people scrub off the odours or douse themselves in perfumes to cover the smells, scientists are desperate to discover how to bottle the scents, known as pheromones, so they can sell it as perfume!

As for shaving, women in Britain and the US do, women in Europe don't, as a rule. Just don't let anyone tell you armpit hair is weird or gross or unusual. Millions of women have free-range armpits.

The parts in your pants It is very important never to put deodorant or perfume, or any kind of douche or spray up into the vagina or onto the genital area.

Your apparatus is self-cleaning on the inside and you can do the rest yourself every day on the outside bits with soap and water and a good rinse. The chemicals in 'feminine hygiene' products can throw out the natural balance of the yeasts and friendly bacteria in your vagina and many people get rashes from using these on such sensitive skin. Yowww.

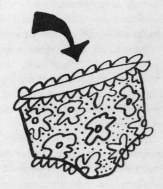

Do I have normal teeth?

Tooth wrangling Think carefully before considering braces. Are they intended to correct a problem with chewing? Because your teeth will last longer if they're not crowding each other out? Because you know it's what you want? Is it a teeny tiny overbite nobody else really notices? Is having them something you may regret later, or have you really thought it through and discussed it with friends and family? Are you doing it just because the dentist says you should, and your parents assume you want it? Are you just temporarily sensitive about your teeth because of a comment from a dork who was trying to make himself feel superior? Could we perhaps put out a contract on the dork instead?

When considering 'bonding' (sounds like what men do on wilderness/percussion camping holidays) to fill a gap between teeth or cover a chip, think about the unique character you might erase from your face. Be aware that the bond itself is more vulnerable to chipping than tooth enamel and find out which foods might stain the bonding materials. Also remember that a chipped tooth may be more vulnerable to decay, and that bonding may stop you feeling self-conscious about smiling. Check whether your bonding is reversible. And be prepared for people not to notice. As in, 'Have you changed your hairstyle or something?'

Never have teeth removed unnecessarily. The natural tooth is always better and less likely to run into trouble if you look after it.

Don't automatically agree to anything: go home and consider your options with the help of pamphlets or photocopied explanations from the surgery and your own notes on prices. Remember that a purely cosmetic treatment can be put off but a long delay in treatment for a health problem in your mouth will almost certainly lead to more pain and costs later on.

Don't be talked into anything cosmetic by a smooth-talking dentist who plays on your insecurities about your smile. Some dentists have a ridiculous chart from the US called a Smile Assessment Chart in which your teeth are rated, and your smile given a score, or even a 'fail'. (Patients should be able to respond with a Dentist's Personality Assessment Chart.) This is nothing but a way of getting you to spend money. It is not scientific and in my opinion you should not go back to a dentist who uses one.

Cosmetic surgery

Who needs it? Cosmetic surgery is not gentle. It's about cutting, slicing, gouging, grasping, pulling, blood, bruising and plastic drains left poking out of wounds to allow fluids to escape from the body after an operation. The bulk of the work is violent, unnecessary surgery on healthy people which is presented more prettily and inaccurately as 'nips and tucks' or 'sculpting'.

Somewhere along the line the bizarre, scary, degrading practice of surgery on normal women gained respectability from the media and writers such as Dr Miriam Stoppard. She refers to the purpose of liposuction as removing 'unsightly bulges such as at the top of thighs and the arms'.

She advises that 'with modern operations and new techniques of cosmetic surgery, it is possible to re-contour almost any part of the body if you are unhappy with the shape you've got...What you have to weigh up is the trade-off: are you the kind of woman who wants to look good in clothes, or do you wish to be free from scars when you are naked?'

Actually, Miriam, old sausage, I'm the kind of woman who doesn't want to undergo general anaesthetic unless I have no choice. I'm the kind of woman who thinks 'cosmetic' surgery is only okay in the most extreme cases – breast reduction to stop back pain, for example. I'm the kind of woman who thinks that your book describing gouging and cutting out bits of arm as 'simple and straightforward' is misleading and an advocacy of mutilation.

Guinea pigs Women have been used as guinea pigs for cosmetic surgery since 1903 when Chicago doctor Charles Miller opened the first cosmetic surgery practice. Miller cut into his customers' bodies and inserted bits of 'braided silk, bits of silk floss, particles of celluloid, vegetable ivory and several other foreign materials' according to his own account of 1926. He returned to general surgery during the Great Depression when demand for cosmetic surgery dropped away.

In the 1920s doctors removed the healthy breasts of women who could not emulate the flat-chested fashion of the day. And all in the name of profit, in the guise of helping women's self-esteem.

Publicity The only recognised experts in the field are plastic surgeons of course and you don't hear much from them about pain (often described as 'discomfort' or 'problems'). Pain, especially extended pain over hours, days and weeks, can have a terrible effect on the body and the mind in physical and psychological shock and distress. The pain, bruising and damage done to the body by many cosmetic surgery operations is comparable to injuries sustained during a car accident.

Newspapers perpetuate the hard sell. Former Australian 'first lady' Hazel Hawke was 'radiant and looking years younger' after her face lift, according to a national magazine: 'Stitches, swelling and pain all but a fading memory.'

Using the Hawke face lift as an example, a newspaper article was more prescriptive. 'Give yourself a lift', said the headline. 'Thinking about a face lift – why not go the whole hog and get a complete make-over?' the article began. 'Those magnificent men with their cutting devices can snip, tuck, tighten, reduce, increase and streamline almost every part of the human body.'

An unnamed surgeon quoted in the article said most of his customers did not have operations because of vanity but because of their 'deformities'. He classed a big nose and small breasts as deformities, adding that a woman with small breasts 'can't wear certain types of clothes. Whenever she is with other women who wear tight T-shirts or clothes and who look a bit feminine, she feels just not feminine.'

The surgeon complained that GPs often sent their patients home who asked for a referral to a plastic surgeon and had to wait for another 'trigger incident' to provoke a more spirited request. 'For example they might have broken up with a boyfriend or separated from a husband or they are under other stresses and they feel this is one stress they want to unload.' Very vulnerable people should be reassured, not cut open.

Magazines often run 'before and after' photographs of surgery. The 'after' photographs are usually taken once the swelling and bruising have faded. There are never 'during' photos or 'straight after' photos or 'two years later' photos.

Amateur hour Cosmeticians, or cosmetic doctors, or 'aesthetic surgeons' may have no specialist training. The British Association of Aesthetic Plastic Surgeons wouldn't recommend anyone to go to private clinics which advertise, as the surgeons there don't have to be properly qualified. 'They only need your permission. Your hairdresser could do it. Anyone.' Members of the British Association of

Aesthetic Plastic Surgeons are not allowed to advertise. So beware of those who do. One woman who had a face lift at a clinic because she saw their advertisement spent £3,500 on a botched job which left her with raised, red scars, eyes that would not close for months, and asymmetrical eyelids.

Although there are lots of adverts recommending surgery, there is no information about the procedure. Pain is not mentioned. There is no pamphlet on reasons not to have surgery, or other options to consider instead of plastic surgery. Almost all the information we have on procedures comes directly from surgeons or clinics, not exactly unbiased sources.

Liposuction Although most surgery brochures do not mention pain, all accounts by liposuction customers do. *Fashion Quarterly* interviewed some of them. 'It hurt like hell for a month,' says one, who says now she's out of proportion because fat has gathered in places it never used to – her waist and knees. 'Now I'm more depressed than I was before I had liposuction, because now that escape route from fatness, which I saved for 18 months to afford, has been taken away from me.' It seems the natural padding had lost its natural home.

She took 'mind-numbing' painkillers. 'It was painful even to walk…I had liposuction to make me look thinner, but I couldn't move so I put on more kilos.' Another woman was left with scarring from the metal tubes stuck through her skin to break up and suck up fat cells.

Another woman, who had liposuction by an internationally renowned surgeon, had ballooned in the torso and waist. 'In my case, I think, the operation unbalanced me for a while, although I don't blame anyone else for that. It was so incredibly painful.' 'If you look at some of the earlier facial liposuction devotees their faces aren't sleek – they're gaunt, skeletonised,' reported the magazine. 'I suffered widespread bruising and couldn't sit down for about three weeks,' said another woman. 'It was a disaster. I ended up using my whole year's holiday to recover.'

A *Mode* reporter wrote of her liposuction. She recalled feeling like a victim of her culture as she dialled the surgeon on the telephone.

'Like most women, I disliked my hips and thighs. Unlike most women, I was lucky enough to have the money to do something about them.' She said that her father had plump hips and her shape is genetic.

'What nobody tells you beforehand is that you're only sedated at the very last moment and you will have to face your doctor and his staff wide awake and naked.' Knocked out, the customer does not hear the grinding, 'gruesome sound' of the liposuction machine or see the operating team shift the body like a piece of meat, 'using your bootee-covered feet as handles'.

She added, 'For the first 12 hours post-op you must urinate about every ten minutes, at a time when sitting down is about as comfortable as swallowing molten lead...I have a fairly high tolerance for pain, but the first few days after surgery I lay on my stomach munching pain killers. For two weeks thereafter I lumbered stiffly to work like Frankenstein, knowing that one careless bump into another human being would make me scream...

'The aching continued, only gradually diminishing, for three months...The seventh week after surgery you're supposed to be able to run. I couldn't, and neither could any of the patients I spoke to. It took ten weeks.' She cited 12 reported liposuction deaths in the US and one woman who was left with a hole in her thigh and haemorrhaging underneath the skin from knee to ankle.

'Standard liposuction,' she said, 'rips out the fat globules through suction and the sheer muscle power of the surgeon.' Next, the reporter wants to have the marks under her eyes cut out. But she's not doing this for her man. 'Two weeks before surgery I met the man I'll probably marry. He liked my hips and thighs the way they were.'

Noses One plastic surgery clinic does nothing to reassure people about their magnificent honkers. They go so far as to recommend deviousness to avoid someone who loves you advising you against a painful, non-medical operation. 'A large or deformed nose can often attract undesirable comment. Ultimately one's self-confidence can erode and personality problems may develop. The modern rhinoplasty is a simple and safe operation which readily overcomes this potential social dilemma [sic]...The fewer people you tell about your proposed operation the better. By all means discuss your operation

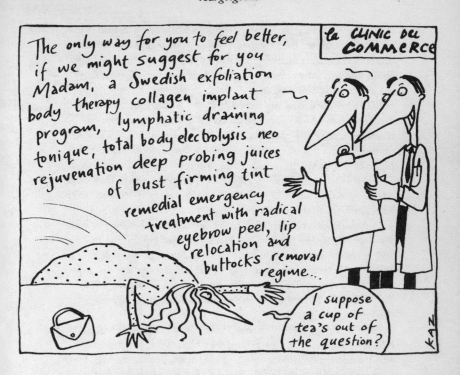

with a close friend, they will be in a position to give you sympathetic and unbiased advice. In contrast to this members of your family who have known you from childhood and, for emotional reasons, are inclined to advise you against having any facial alterations.' Oh, emotional reasons, like love. Pah. Pass the scalpel, sweetie.

The breast business explained

By a conservative estimate, at least two million American women have had breast implants.

Fake breasts are now made from a liquid saline (salt) filler contained in a solid bag made from the same stuff they use for replacement heart valves. You know why? Because so many women have sued the makers of the previous breast filling, silicone, which is a close chemical relative to Silly Putty.

For years, women have told stories of hardening, lumpy breasts, silicone lumps moving up under armpits and rupturing during mammography tests for breast cancer. Implants also make it harder to detect breast cancer, the biggest cancer killer of women. The saline-liquid implants, encased in a rubbery shell made of silicone, carry a risk of deflation and leaking.

Medical journalists predicted that the leaking of the silicone implants would cause immune problems. And so it came to pass. It is now estimated that there have been many breakages and leakages from silicone implants and that, in those women, anecdotal evidence supports disruption to the immune system. 'It is well established,' reported Dr Ronald Laura in *Nature and Health* magazine, that 'small amounts of silicone fluid seep from all silicone gel implants, even when they are not ruptured'.

One young woman who had breast implants at the age of 18 went through hell as they ruptured and leaked, causing pain and anxiety, and another operation to remove some of the bags. She still has the pain that started after the rupturing. 'I feel like ripping out my spine,' she said. 'I want to tell girls who are thinking of getting implants [that] we should stay the way we're born and not have anything artificial in us.

'You're vulnerable as a teenager and you want to look your best. But when you have something like this, you can't go back.' Manuafacturers of silicone implants told women that the bags were inert and would last a lifetime, but then proceeded to set aside over £2 billion to compensate women with implants. An unnecessary precaution to take if they truly believed in their product?

Thousands of women have had silicone implants. Several of them, desperate for help, turned to support groups to share stories, information and legal advice. One woman tried to remove her own implants with a razor; several tried suicide. The Women's Implant Network fought to have doctors agree to give implants back to their patients when removed so they could be inspected.

The lonely and vulnerable position of women patients in the medical system is poignantly illustrated by the women who pinned little notes on their surgical gowns to be read when they were unconscious, asking for their implants back.

By August 1993, when it was reported, manufacturers admitted that tests on rats showed silicone to be a strong irritant to the immune system, but did not accept that this could necessarily be applied to

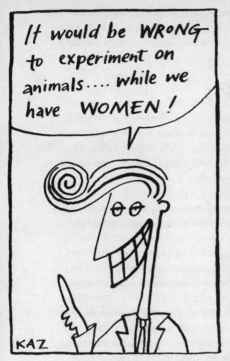

It would be WRONG to experiment on animals.... while we have WOMEN!

KAZ

humans. Soon after, a Californian study found that one-third of women with implants had a measurable immune system reaction. This seems to make sense: a foreign unnatural object in the body surely must have an effect on the part of the body's system which detects and fights foreign bodies and viruses.

The medical director of the Centre for Immune, Environmental and Toxic Disorders in Texas said there was evidence that children of women with silicone implants had developed silicone antibodies, showing that the silicone had entered and altered their immune systems. All 60 children he studied had abnormal immune systems. The control group of kids whose mothers had natural breasts had normal variations to their immune systems.

Another US doctor said kids breastfed by silicone-implanted breasts demonstrated symptoms similar to a muscle-wasting disease which occurs more frequently in women with implants. One mother with the disease had a seven-year-old son who started showing the same symptoms. 'The doctors tell me I'm mad,' she said. 'I feel like there is a heated rod in there burning my spine.' The woman has had three operations – silicone implants, saline implant replacement and saline implant removal.

And still the propaganda comes. On the front cover of one magazine in August/September 1993, 'scar free surgery' was announced. By the time you got to the story, the 'revolutionary new [sic] breast-lift technique' was said to 'minimise' scarring. A closer read predicted 'faint' scarring. Saline implants in a silicone shell would be used. The last two paragraphs of the report noted that some lifting with the upper body (what other part of the body is used for lifting?) was out of the question forever after the operation, and there was a risk of the knot from the stitching inside the breast becoming twisted and feeling like a lump.

Collagen implants Collagen, fat from cows collected in the blood and din of an abattoir, is injected under the skin, usually to make a fat lip, also known as Paris Lip, or Oh My God Have You Run Into A Door Handle? It costs about from £350 per syringe and can also be injected into wrinkles to plump them out.

A test patch is always done first to check for any allergy. Usually the collagen is injected into the arm, and they'll charge you more than £80 for it. If there is no reaction after a month, the service is performed.

The effect is temporary. The body absorbs all the collagen within two to six months. In April 1992, *Cleo* magazine reported that the US Food and Drug Administration made collagen manufacturers put a warning on their product that customers who have auto-immune disorders should not use it. Collagen manufacturers maintain that cow collagen cannot cause the human immune system to attack itself, so it cannot start an auto-immune problem. There is no long-term study on the effects of animal collagen used in this way.

The surgeons Cosmetic surgeon Dr Darryl Hodgkinson told a magazine that he was initially sceptical about laser surgery. The first lasers, he said, were 'massive and not that easy to control'. Also, they heated the surrounding skin up so much there was a lot of charred tissue.'

Another thing Dr Hodgkinson didn't like was the fact that customers – people – bruised. 'One of the problems in our work is morbidity, the swelling and bruising patients experience after surgery. We do everything we possibly can – select patients carefully, get them off aspirin, talk to them about proper nutrition, "ice" them on the table – but still they bruise.' He became convinced that laser surgery could reduce bruising.

But the body will bruise if you hurt it. That's what it's for, it's the body's way of recovering after an injury. It's an injury that plastic surgeons might call 'treatment'. *Elle* magazine also reported that six cases have been reported of customers being incinerated by lasers. In Australia, lasers can be used by doctors untrained in their use. This apparent danger to customers is opposed by the Royal College of Surgeons, which would like to restrict laser surgery to specifically trained doctors, not just any bozo with a laser machine.

A specifically trained bozo is another matter entirely.

Dr Leo Rozner, an accredited plastic surgeon, and no bozo, likens his practice to virtual reality. He says, 'The technology is available and the pressures of fashion and compliance influence people. They can see the ideal face any day on television. It's rubbish that surgeons use their patients. The patients ask for what they want and they must be fully informed and research the matter. We are fixing deformities. Surgeons won't touch on schizoids or dysmorphics [people who are obsessed with tiny parts of themselves].' But the *Oxford Dictionary* defines 'deform' as what Dr Rozner is paid to do: 'To make ugly, deface; put out of shape, misshape.'

Dr Rozner suggests, 'We cannot advertise, so we have to tell the truth.' On the subject of breasts, he says, 'Boobs go in and out of fashion but I have had a suit for 20 years and it has been in fashion three times. It depends what's happening but it can give women confidence and acceptability. Some are happy with the porky look.'

He is unhappy with the media image of plastic surgeons. 'We are reputable. We don't do anything without informed consent. The demands and the technology are growing in leaps and bounds. Melbourne has had its share of disasters [he named a cosmetic surgeon who killed a few customers with botched liposuction] but the technology is like a Mercedes. You don't get a 12-year-old to drive it.'

He advises customers to look at the doctor's track record (I suppose you could knock on the door of his previous customers and demand to see their nipples) and build up a rapport with the doctor in time, before deciding. 'There are risks of course. You buy a car and there are no guarantees that you won't have an accident. Never do business with a person you don't like, whether it's second-hand cars or second-hand faces,' he says.

I do not suggest that all plastic surgeons are disreputable or sneaky

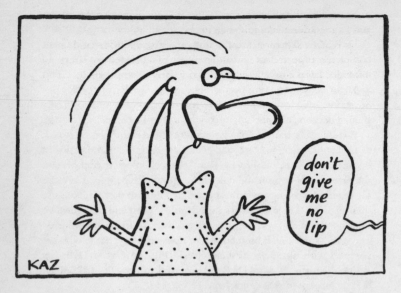

or that they cajole customers into unwanted operations, although I am quite sure these things have happened. I do suggest that somebody who talks about the 'porky' look, who compares women's bodies to suits and cars, and medical procedures to a Mercedes, is not a person I care to agree with. I found Dr Rozner to be honest, helpful and charming. But he too believes that women are 'deformed' by the natural process of ageing, or if they have small breasts. I think that sucks.

In his 'Avenue Cosmetic Plastic Surgery Health Update' newsletter to customers, Dr Rozner describes a person's cosmetic surgery as a job prerequisite. 'It is now part of the investment in their work, rather like dressing up for the office. It is also an investment in themselves as their prestige and success in employment are importantly and closely linked with their looks. You never, ever get a second chance to make a good impression at a job interview.'

His brochure offers, 'If desired, Asian features can be softened by enlarging the nose and making it narrower, by reducing the flare of the nostrils and by lifting the bridge of the nose to make it a more prominent feature. A double eyelid can be achieved by reducing skin and fat to make the fold higher,' and, 'we aim for excellence and occasionally achieve perfection.' One can only hope that Asian girls and women don't take this seriously.

Dr Rozner says surgery can improve a person's image, and seems completely unaware of the chilling nature of his statement, 'In many instances, facial cosmetic surgery is psychiatry with a knife.'

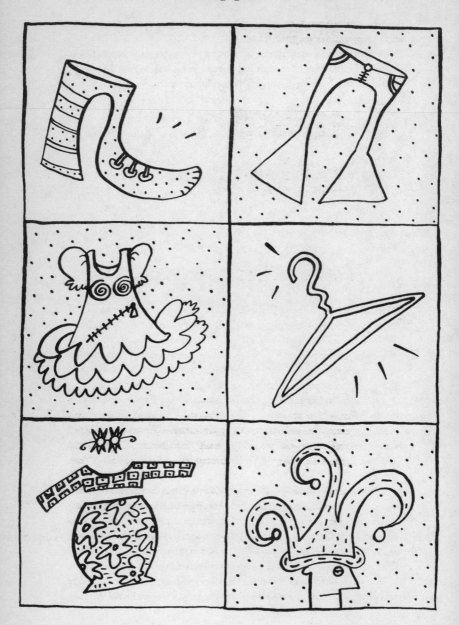

chapter *four*

Fashion victims

Models and role models

Heroines Books and magazines for girls have always been full of role models: some interesting, some blindingly tedious. Girls' annuals, a staple reading diet for girls until about the 1960s, were always full of daring schoolgirls catching smugglers or solving crimes, or exploring vast, 'unexplored' wildernesses otherwise quite familiar to the indigenous people, or slaughtering another team at hockey.

Not that I'm suggesting that we should all go back to reading books about Millicent of the Upper Fourth – far too many secret midnight eating binges in the dorms, for a start – but at least there were some roles for women. They actually *did* things. They didn't just stand around looking at the camera trying to sell you an A-line frock.

Now our role models are more likely to be presented as simply silent, involved in nothing more challenging than pouting, or riding a bike, as long as it's just to tone up the thighs and not necessarily to *go* anywhere. Books for teenage girls are often just about how to find a guy (or how to lose one and get another). Models may be smart, funny women, but that's not why they're famous.

We have to find our own role models by discovering books with real heroines, movies about feisty women, stories of girls and women who do more than drape themselves over half a palm tree in a £200 bikini.

Magazines point out the different definitions of beauty we have for actresses and models. They have freckles and gaps in their teeth and they range from brunettes to blondes, with short hair or long. We are told that there is far more individuality now than there used to be. But look at what all those varied faces do have in common. Overwhelmingly they're white and, even more overwhelmingly, they are all carried by thin bodies. They don't reflect all of us. It is the same for soapie stars, for newsreaders, for almost any woman allowed onto our screens.

American film actress Andie McDowell says, 'They only want you if you have a voice like a woman, a body like a girl and a mind like a man...If one more person asks me to lose five pounds, I'm going to be sick. I don't want to go through it any more and I don't want my daughter to go through it either. We've made some progress, but not much.'

The images of women and girls that we see on television are completely censored. Any woman photographed for a magazine is photographed with a lot of make-up, usually a photographer with a brief to flatter her and, in the case of American magazines, often a retouch job as well. Very often, famous people have a power of veto over which photographs of themselves are used. Authors usually choose their own publicity photographs (I personally destroyed the one of me wearing only a singlet on the bunny rug).

The associate photo editor of a famous American celebrity magazine in New York won't give celebrities power of veto but she will ask them what they're worried about and look out for it herself, including 'lines on their neck or whatever'. The editor, who wants to remain anonymous, says most things are taken care of in the *two hours* usually allotted for hair and make-up before the photography begins. She feels that retouching a photograph if a chin looks weird because of the way the light hits it is no different from setting up lights in the first place. 'It's just another phase in the whole thing, and it's not real. None of it is real.'

She can remember the time a famous rock star had her armpits made up and she trusted her personal make-up artist so much she didn't bother looking in the mirror when he was finished. 'He was completely transforming her face...accentuating the eyes, the cheekbones and all that stuff but to a much greater degree, which looks kind of weird in person, but on film it works.' And the cost?

'Probably the more run-of-the-mill portrait without too much of an entourage is about £1000, depending on how much everybody charges. The photographers make the most money.

> The boys at my school are just waiting for the next Elle Macpherson to walk through the door. One guy even collects Elle memorabilia and had a scrapbook with her pictures in it. The boys are 14 to 15-ish and very immature. They will wake up when they realise the shortage of Elles in this world. Why can't we have healthy role models of all sizes, so it's fair to everyone? Why does everyone have this Beauty Thing? It is like a curse and eventually wrecks people's lives.
>
> Kelly, 14

'One of the things I find interesting is how you have this really long time to do hair and make-up and there doesn't look like there is any on, you know there's a *lot* of make-up but it's so…it's an illusion. All it's done has changed something, but you can't put your finger on it. It's a painting, it's truly a painting at that point. One make-up guy works with many divas: he paints. It's not like you or I would put lipstick on.

'The other thing that's interesting is when you go ohhh, they've really messed them up, they've got so much make-up on they look like shit and then in the photographs it doesn't look like that, it just looks like they're beautiful…you don't put make-up on men, you might put a little bit, but mostly what you do with a guy is you'll just put a bit of powder on them so there is no shine in the lights. And then the hair gets done.' Later, changes may be made to the photographs on computer screen.

> TV and magazines: to me, I see all those gorgeous models and I think, 'Wow. She's got a great bod! I wish!'
>
> Sal, 19

Coathangers These days, the beauty-contest replacement seems to be cover-girl contests where young girls aspire to be models or disembodied, disembrained 'faces of the year'. These contests are often sponsored by model agencies who help choose the winner and then start making money out of her. Being a model is almost always presented as something glamorous and exciting and wonderful.

Only about 5 to 10 per cent of women are in the height and weight range of models. Most models are 5ft 7 tall and wear size 10 or 12 dress with unusually wide shoulders, bust size 32 to 34-in, bra cup A or B, waist 25 to 26-in and hips 34 to 36-in. Models must also have unusually wide shoulders. Cindy Crawford is about two stone lighter than the average woman of her height: over 5ft 8 and size eight. 'I think women see me on the cover of magazines and think I never have a pimple or bags under my eyes,' says Ms Crawford. 'You have to realise that's after two hours of hair and make-up, plus (photo) retouching. Even *I* don't wake up looking like Cindy Crawford.'

A reporter at the New York fashion collections looks at the women on the catwalks and concludes, 'There are no thighs in sight – it's hard to believe these women are the same species as me, let alone the same gender'.

Somewhere along the line, the thin girls who had shoulders like coathangers became not just models but 'supermodels' and, even more puzzling, role models. They are asked for beauty hints, opinions and space-filling quotes. None of this is memorable unless it is arrogant ('We don't get out of bed for less than $10,000 a day,' said Linda Evangelista) or stupid. (Asked why there are no books in her apartment, Elle Macpherson said, 'I don't think you should read what you haven't written'.) None of it is important because of what is being said, only because of who is saying it.

Ms Macpherson, called 'The Body' by the media as if there were only one, and called a role model because she's rich, produces calendars that are nothing more than soft porn: nipples and cleavages straining and swimsuits to emphasise not sporting achievement but a very unusual body shape. Elle Macpherson's calendars, like the 'dirty postcards' of days gone by and *Playboy* magazines, serve a dual purpose. They're for men to admire and hide under their mattresses and for girls and women to use as some sort of unattainable, forever-crushing goal – even though getting a body like that without the right genes is impossible. (Soon after I wrote this Ms Macpherson went the whole hog and posed for *Playboy* anyway.)

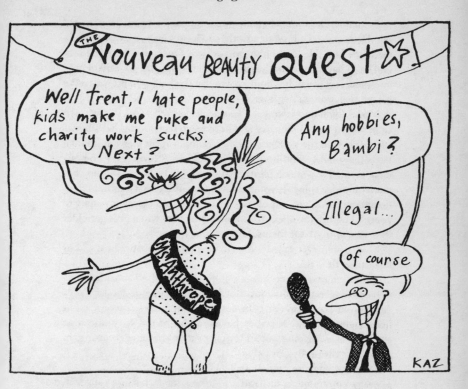

This year's models Almost all models are told what to wear, what to do with their hair, how to look, how to act, what kind of an image to project – in short, what kind of a person they are. Models are 'managed', treated like children, possibly because some of them are. Models are, excuse the language, treated like shit.

The truth is, models are some of the most insecure, tortured souls around. The industry likes them that way. They're more likely to always do what they're told: look blank or perky. Perkily blank, maybe. Or blankly perky. That's about the range.

Many models *are* smart. It's just that their job does not reward them for it.

At an American model convention, one agent wants 15-year-old skin for cosmetics ads while another addresses girls in a queue waiting to see him. He likes only 'one or two. One and a half. The second half I have talk to my plastic surgeon.' The girl, 15, will be told by a model agency in her home town that she has no future unless she has an operation on her nose.

Model Lynn Snowden told *Esquire* magazine, 'Models have such an obsession with minor flaws. The average receptionist has a better self-image than the average model.' A model agent explains how he treats the women who keep him in business. 'Never, ever compliment them. They're complimented constantly by losers. It's sick, but this is an inside thing. If you mention something that's an imperfection about them, say, a mole, or their hair looks bleached – they're yours.' Another top agent told a magazine that when girls get older they start to think for themselves too much.

Models are never called women; only girls, no matter how old or how smart they are.

It must be easy to get things out of proportion when eating anything at all is seen as some kind of weakness. Teenage model Tanya Arpadi told a magazine that she loves food and doesn't worry about her weight. Yet she describes having a cup of tea and some toast after school as 'pigging out'. Her only other reference to eating, in front of the telly, is also described as 'pigging out'. It is as if any consumption of food at all is presented as greed.

Lingerie modelling is better paid than other modelling jobs and many models get breast implants to do it. Inevitably, the models themselves, as individuals, cop it from the press, even from a magazine which once idolised them. 'The pumped up hair and breasts and stature of

> I open a magazine and a supermodel stares back at me, her waist the size of a Polo mint. An article accompanying the picture constantly mentions how beautiful she is. I immediately drop the magazine and start doing sit-ups. Can you blame me?
>
> Sarah

[the 1980s supermodels] symbolises the excesses of the 1980s,' said one magazine. Another called the waifs 'snotty stringbeans in their skimpy, wimpy threads'.

Magazines now run stories on models as they used to on movie stars. One has a regular tear-out double postcard of a male and female model in each issue. Obviously, the obsession with models is selling magazines. We learn from lists of their characteristics in *Cosmopolitan* that 'virtues' include 'always keeps her skin looking perfect', 'avoids partying', and 'doesn't drink coffee'. Vices include 'chocolates and croissants', 'ice-cream', 'junk food', 'a tendency to flirt' and 'sweet foods'. Eating and flirting! Vices! Give me a break!

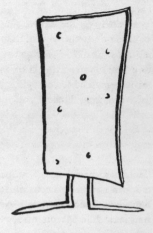

waifer - thin

The make-up job on models

'*Harper's Bazaar* retouches photographs of girls like crazy. Other magazines too. They just take out any imperfections. They'll slim a girl's hips or lengthen her legs. They can do anything now,' a New York make-up artist says. 'When you're doing their make-up you can see...like they're really heavy under the eyes, really dark, and the girls who have lines around their eyes and you see the picture (in the magazine) and it's completely smooth, or maybe their eyes were bloodshot that day, the eyes are real bright and white. It's amazing what you can do even [with make-up].'

The endless cycle

The first fashion parade models, in London in 1900, were all tall and big. None of them weighed less than 11 stone, and 'several of them considerably more'.

Lately models are tall and thin. Big breasts are sometimes 'fashionable', sometimes not.

In the 1960s the first waifs were personified by Penelope Tree and Twiggy (Lesley Hornby). In the early 1990s they were Kate

Moss and Australian Emma Balfour. Kate Moss, at less than seven and a half stone and 5ft 6 tall is unusually short for modelling and underweight by all health and medical guidelines. But she has coathanger shoulders. Magazine editors called the waifs the 'cut-price models', those who work for thousands of dollars less than their predecessors in their eagerness to become as well known.

> I also feel pressure from magazines. They advertise clothes for people maybe 15 and up, but they use these 12, 13-year-old models who haven't even started puberty yet. How are we supposed to compete with girls who have boys' bodies?
>
> Melissa, 15

Emma Balfour says she sometimes worries about the effect waif-worship has on young girls. 'When I feel fat I don't eat so much,' this very skinny girl told *Who Weekly*.

Those in the industry seem to want to have it both ways: the bigger models make women feel better about themselves, but the waifs have no effect at all. Richard Harper, director of Cameron's actors and models agency in Australia, says he is violently against the waif look. Elle Macpherson, he said, 'served as a catalyst. Suddenly girls could have a shape.' Later in the same interview he said women do not change to suit fashion. 'I don't take responsibility for any of it and what's more I've never yet met a woman who'd do anything I wanted her to do.'

Harper's Bazaar ran a seven-page feature claiming that the waifs were so thin only because of genes and hard work. Penelope Tree says she was a miserable anorexic at the height of her period of fame and adulation as a '60s waif model. In some photographs of her at the time, she looks remarkably like Kate Moss, the same hollow cheeks and dull eyes – and indeed designer Calvin Klein says he first booked Moss because she reminded him of Penelope Tree, more 'real' than the bigger supermodels.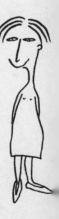

Harper's Bazaar defended its use of the waif models against outraged letters from readers. 'What you're seeing on our pages is not a horde of starvation-riven women. This is an ectomorphic body type. It's in fashion…Eating disorders are not new complaints. People were dieting long before newsstands were invented.'

Cleo was horrified and called it 'the fashion look that should carry a health warning…They might be in, but at what cost?…The blank-slate waifs of the 1990s, with their empty, childlike attitude, are helplessness personified. The look may be 1970s grunge, but the message is pure 1950s helplessness.'

Allure magazine cited the waifs as 'the triumph of poverty, of vulnerability'. Kate Moss's photographer Corinne Day said, 'I love reality – things like bad posture, vacant stares, skinniness.' (Drug addiction, war, famine, tennis anybody?) Dress designer Valentino said, 'I love these young, new girls, frail and insecure.' (Creep.) *Harper's Bazaar* concluded, 'Like to be Kate Moss? We all would.' Speak for yourself.

> I try to like myself for what I am but I open up a magazine and immediately compare myself with those perfect models.
>
> Jacquiline, 17

US modelling agent Eileen Ford sneers at the very idea that the idealisation of models might have a bad influence. 'Models do not have a negative impact on women. They have a positive impact because they set standards. Women are going to look like themselves but they will look like their best selves because models set standards. When you think you look your best, and feel your best there's an aura around you of self-confidence and self-assurance. Models do that to women.' What models did to one reporter at the New York fashion shows in 1993, she said, was make her feel 'fat and malformed all week'.

It was reported that the bigger models were dieting to be even thinner, to compete. The thinner models make the others feel scared. A New York make-up artist told me of working on a shoot with a well-known model. 'The day I worked with her, all day long she was hungry, so hungry. I said, well, eat something, do you want me to get you a bagel or something? "No, no, no, I can't eat, I can't eat, I can't eat. I can't work if I eat." And that was just crazy. She finally had a sip of orange juice at four o'clock. She's so thin, so thin…I think a lot of them do drugs because I don't think there's any way you can be that thin without doing something. I have seen lots of photographs of [a famous model] when she had got really anorexic but a lot of the time they are dressed and you don't really see it. Her waist was the size of my thigh, probably thinner.'

The make-up artist said she sometimes has to camouflage the skin of a waif. 'I tend to give them colour so they look more alive. Sort of like a heroin addict…when you are that thin it's hard to keep your skin good, you need lots of aids.'

Diane Parks, the Australian editor of *Slimming* magazine, says: '[Fashion photography] is like food photography, you tart it up a bit because you don't have the other things that go with real food, like taste and smell. With pictures of models, you don't get those other parts about meeting human beings, like personality.'

> Whenever I open magazines I look at the models. They are so lucky to have a perfect body and perfect skin. Like the girls on the pictures advertising L'Oreal products. I recently had this guy kissing me and all that stuff that happens and haven't heard from him since. It totally sux.
>
> Lottie, 14

Tortured models Models rarely admit to having eating disorders until their modelling careers are over. *Who Weekly* ran a cover story called 'The Price of Beauty', a story of 'supermodels' Carol Alt, Beverly Johnson and Kim Alexis, in which the three women detailed their low self-esteem, 'nightmare diets' and 'vicious treatment on the job'. Success meant 'a constant gnawing hunger'. 'They met the enemy and it was food.' The healthy image was attained with lighting, make-up and a public brainwashed to believe that thin was always healthy.

Kim Alexis said the head of Elite Modelling agency 'guaranteed me a certain amount of money if I lost a stone'. Carol Alt was a straight-A student when a photographer noticed her. The first agent she contacted 'told me I'd be perfect if I lost a stone'.

Ms Alexis says, 'I remember trying every fad diet. I remember starving myself for four days in a row.' She shared a flat with model Kelly Emberg. 'One night I was eating only a head of lettuce for dinner. Kelly walked in and said, "You're eating a *whole* head of lettuce? How could you?" I cried and said "But it's all I've had all day. It's not even 50 calories".'

'I think I was a normal person before I started screwing around with these diets. My metabolism got screwed up. I lost my period for

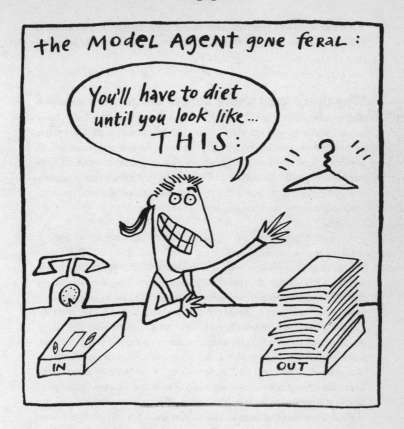

two full years…I'd dread lunch because the client would look at me [during a shoot] and say, "You're not going to eat that are you?"'

Carol Alt says, 'Do you remember the Beverly Hills diet? You only ate fruit. It was terrible. At another point I was drinking eight cups of coffee a day and I ate salad for dinner. On my first modelling job I fainted. An editor had given me one month to lose 10 pounds. If I did she promised me a trip to Rome…So I stopped eating. Maybe I'd have celery, an apple. I went along doing the one salad a night routine for a year. I remember feeling so tired and depressed. I had no personal life…eventually I learned to eat five small meals a day'.

'In our profession clothes look better on a hanger, so you have to look like a clothes hanger. It will never change,' said Beverly Johnson.

Why don't they show bigger models? It seems that

magazines only use size 10 models because the designers and manufacturers only give them size 10 samples to photograph. The magazine editors do not challenge this, and a stereotype is maintained.

But the real reason why models are size 10 has nothing to do with what is acceptable in real life and *everything* to do with all the money to be made by the fashion industry, which still calls the shots, provides the samples, and creates an atmosphere of envy to help sell their product.

Carlotta Moye, fashion editor of *Dolly* magazine says, 'We are working a season ahead and there is only one sample...We had a 15-year-old on a photo shoot and she put on half a stone on the trip and the pictures just did not look good – she put it on in the boobs and hips and she lost her aspirational appeal. We had to crop the picture below the waist...She has lost it now and she's back to her perfect self – she only just got her period a few months ago.

'There isn't just one body shape in the magazines – things change. I don't go for weight when I choose models, I go for personality. Weight ranks maybe third or fourth on the list of requirements. Sometimes we get letters saying models look too skinny. Some people say we should make her look fatter. Women are very critical and bitchy. They never criticise hair colour but they are obsessed with weight.'

According to *Vogue* Australia fashion editor Victoria Collison, 'Clothes look better on those small-size girls. You are presenting a look, an image...Clothes can look good on most sized models though. Every May–June we do a working women's story, the strong career women with clothes to fit them – larger than size 8 or 10 – it is a more realistic image, and this is the way we can cover it. The size 10 thing has always happened that way. These clothes could look just as good on a size 14 if she is tall. A magazine has a certain amount of fantasy.'

Girlfriend fashion editor Catherine Murphy says, 'We try to avoid the skinny look if we can because we are aware of the anorexia issue but I think the illness itself is more complex than just the image thing.

With fashion there is a lot of choice now, girls are wearing more boys' clothes. We usually do two stories with bigger and smaller girls. Our readers are younger and slightly smaller anyway. Obviously models are thin and personally I feel strongly about the anorexia issue. Society wants to see them this way [size 10] – that is what the girls want; [size] 14 to 16 is not what they perceive as attractive. Designers see that their garments look better on proportionately thin, taller models.'

'Aspirational appeal' – the atmosphere of envy – seems to be the key here. Fashion editors are choosing what they think we want to be. While the designers are the only ones who will provide the sample clothes and buy the fashion ads in magazines, nothing much will change unless magazine readers *en masse* demand a change. Unsurprisingly perhaps, given their jobs, most fashion editors do not question the notion that different body shapes can be 'in fashion' while the shape of real people stays pretty much the same for each individual.

So, if we want bigger models in the magazines, we have to write and tell them. 'Dear Editor, the model on page 72 of your latest issue looks like a sick whippet. I want to know what the clothes will look like on a size fourteen. And PS, please give that model some lunch before she faints. Signed, Reasonably Outraged Come to Think About It.'

I don't know whether I should stay with the muscly toned look or the waif look. Sometimes I wish supermodels didn't exist and body shape didn't matter because then you wouldn't have to keep up. Since I got weighed in P.E. class everyone, including the teacher, thinks I'm extremely underweight and no one wants to help me with a diet. Why doesn't someone help me with a healthy diet that will help me lose weight and make me look like one of those models? Because I know I'd feel better about myself if I did.

Anonymous

My boyfriend has supermodels all over his walls, which is a little annoying, but he always reassures me.

Lena, 19

145

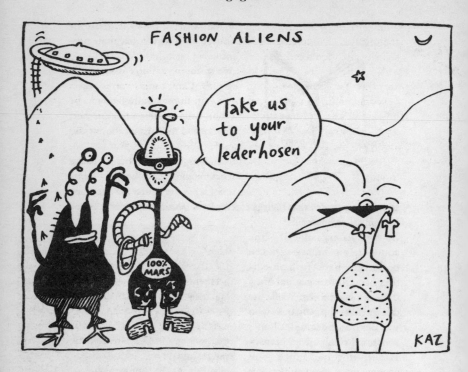

The fashion industry

Girly lures Women's fashion chain-stores have been made into one-stop girly lures, offering everything under the one roof: shoes, undies, accessories, hairclips, jewellery. Each store tries to create an image, a readymade made-up lifestyle. Some have pop music interspersed with ads for products in the shop broadcast continuously and blow-up photographs of models, often with accessories, including a boyfriend (not in stock). The shops provide casual clothes, going-out clothes and work clothes.

Then there are the designer shops with higher price tags and often better cuts, fabrics and more carefully finished clothes. But not always. Women are encouraged by advertising and image-making to choose a designer or two and stick with them: to have a look created for them, rather than finding clothes that go with their look, their personality and their activities.

It is relatively easy to track general fashion. Fashion is generally worn by the young: people in their teens and early twenties who have the money to change their wardrobe and are more likely to be bothered by what others think of them. Style is different altogether: a personal style that suits the personality and pursuits of the wearer and is not dictated by anybody else.

In 1992 total turnover for the British fashion, leather and footwear industries was estimated at £12.5 billion. The number of people employed is falling constantly, due to the government policies that allow unrestricted importing of clothes from overseas, which is cheaper because the people making them are paid about threepence and a sardine a month.

According to one television series about the fashion industry, it's about a three quarters of a trillion pounds a year industry worldwide. Now, I can't be exactly sure what a trillion is, but it's a lot of pocket money and a deposit on a very nice apartment in New York. It's a million billion, or a few squillion. A lot, anyway.

> You always see in movies a perfect guy and a beautiful woman making out anywhere they please. They aren't at all realistic, the women always have beautiful clothes, not just shorts and a T-shirt: matching undies and bras, not the cheap ones where the elastic or wire is falling out!
>
> Tina, 16

So the clothes shops are competing with each other to get you to buy their clothes. They will do this by telling you through their ads and magazines that you *need* their clothes.

Casual wear makes up a large percentage of clothes sold, a trend that will continue with the trend of people working from home. The companies that sell ritzier clothes are finding it hardest to survive. As one fashion buyer put it, 'With the decline of a lot of our (business) entrepreneurs, the market for the £1000 to £1,500 garment has dropped away quite seriously.' Or fairly hilariously, depending on how you look at it.

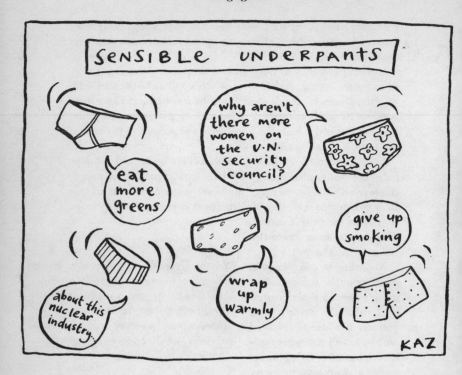

The boom boom Lately (not that you wouldn't have noticed, dear, pass the turnip) we have been having a recession. For instance, bra sales dropped by about a quarter between 1991 and 1992, just when we were being told there was a huge boom in lingerie. Mind you, we are told every year that there's a boom in lingerie. My definition of a boom is not a 24.3 per cent drop in sales, but this is possibly the reason I am not in marketing. There seems to be only a boom in booms, if you know what I mean.

Fashion manufacturers create the styles then try to convince us to buy them. This is why everything changes so dramatically from one season to the next – fluorescent colours one summer, sandy, mushroomy colours the next, so one bit won't match the rest the next time you buy something.

One way manufacturers try and boost sales is the self-proclaimed

> Jennifer: 'So today I'm joined by Dawn French, top fashion expert to the stars and the high street. So tell me, Dawn, what can we expect to see in the shops this year?'
> Dawn: 'Clothes mostly…and some hats and some shoes.'
>
> Comedians Jennifer Saunders and Dawn French

boom, that staple tactic of the lingerie industry promoters. They've been doing it since at least 1952 when National Corset Week was announced. Recently a manufacturer claimed that women were rushing to buy inflatable bras with a little attachment like a bike pump. Oh, say it ain't so!

For a few years now, spurred on by Madonna's conical, comical boosies jutting out from a designer corset, manufacturers have been trying to sell us thousands of 'bustiers': a new-fashioned corset, only slightly more comfy than the whalebone and rubber monstrosities of the past that had women fainting, in floods of sweat and with internal damage. When *Allure* magazine did a fashion spread on them, even the fashion writer had to admit 'It took six hands, all pulling in different directions, to fit the actress [*actress*!!?] photographed here in three bustiers by Valentino. And the largest waist was an enviable 25 inches,' she wrote, betraying only her own envy. She continued, 'there is probably nothing more beautiful than the contours of bare shoulders and barely concealed breasts.' That woman should take a holiday somewhere where you can get scenery.

The Lee jeans company responded cleverly to the piffle about bustiers with a series of ads aimed at real women. 'Corsets. Girdles. High heels. Isn't it time women's clothes were designed for women?' the ad headline implored. The copy continued, 'How could any sane woman, for example, no matter how proud of her torso, have possibly dreamed up the bustier? What about the girdle [named after the sound you make when you try to put one on.]…since women come in different shapes, there are several fits of…jeans available to women…[including] relaxed fit jeans and loose fit. Try finding a relaxed fit corset.'

It is said that Marie Antoinette invented the idea of pushing her bosoms up somewhere around her chin in a low-cut frock, and she certainly didn't have much else to do. Ungaro, a designer, 'invented' a body suit which exposed all of the back, and (I'm about to be indelicate, turn the page if you are easily shocked, thank you) what is politely known as the buttock cleft, otherwise as the bum crack.

Designers who show bosom-twisting cleavage, creating and exposing business suits and botty-exposing jumpsuits cannot seriously expect us to wear it.

The publicity game What they are doing is getting the pictures of their models in the fashion magazines and on the television. The more shocking and, whoopsie there's a nipple, outrageous the better. Almost any publicity is good publicity. Perhaps only two copies of that ridiculous frock exist but many more copies of the photo do.

There, in the magazine, a pouting 15-year-old with a long slash of dark purple on each eyebrow, is wearing an open hospital gown, with an old garbage bag held together with a bulldog clip wrapped around her chest. She is wearing a pair of shorts made from muslin stapled to an old wheat sack. Nobody will ever wear it again. The model certainly wouldn't be seen dead in it unless she were getting paid £1000 for the day.

But the designer has made a splash in an industry where there must be something *new* every minute. The designer's other collection, called 'ready to wear' will indeed be more 'wearable' and copied by factory owners in South East Asia. We'll get a watered-down version of it by spring, and an ad with a picture of a happy young girl wearing it, who is oblivious to the clothes and with her arm around a *boyfriend* (pause for round of applause).

When there are see-through clothes for the office on the catwalk, and the designers suggest long, tight skirts with scarily high heels for women who have to use public transport to get home, we know most people won't really buy them. Manufacturers have tried sever-

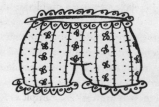

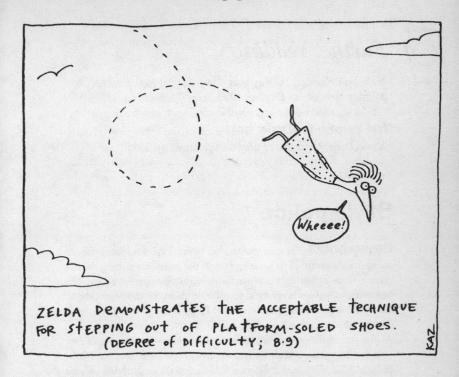

ZELDA DEMONSTRATES THE ACCEPTABLE TECHNIQUE
FOR STEPPING OUT OF PLATFORM-SOLED SHOES.
(DEGREE of DIFFICULTY; 8·9)

al times since the 1960s to bring back the 'baby doll' dress for grown ups and adolescents: it is very rarely seen except in advertisements and the pages of the magazines. Oh, and on baby dolls.

Scary shoes If you must wear high heels, don't wear them every day. They are a known cause or encourager of hammer toes, bunions, corns and lower leg and back problems. Most women don't develop these foot and related problems until their late teens when they start wearing high heels. High heels put two-and-a-half times more weight onto some of the bones in the foot than if you were barefoot. Constant wearing of high heels causes the achilles tendon to shrink, and then when you switch to smaller heels or sport shoes, it can be very painful. Platform shoes are completely stupid.

Further reading

Nicholas Coleridge, *The Fashion Conspiracy: A Remarkable Journey through the Empires of Fashion* (Heinemann, 1988). A fabulously entertaining and well-written book which exposes how the whole thing really works.

Alison Lurie, *Language of Clothes* (Bloomsbury, 1992).

Style police

Bossy boots The style police don't even have a uniform we can recognise them by. (This is only one of the infuriating things about them.) They might be wearing some frightfully expensive tweedy togs with batwing sleeves or a wee bit of cheesecloth draped about their private parts, but they have one thing in common: they think they are the boss of us.

The style police tell us what we should wear – as a matter of fact what we *must* wear and also what we are not allowed to wear. I'll be the first to admit there are clothes I think should be dropped off in a bottomless quarry on Saturn. But there *are* people who like to wear lime green stretch polyester and orange A-line frocks, and good luck to them.

The style police think that what we look like is more important than anything (*particularly* world peace) and it is their job to seek out and punish those who break their own fashion rules. Some of them are obviously stupid: 'I consider that without hats, an intrinsic part of fashion, we would have no civilisation,' said dressmaker and dillbrain Christian Dior in 1957.

And therein lies a clue to why the style police behave in such a way. There are many different squads in the style police. There are designers, sellers and advertisers of clothes who will make money out of selling an 'essential' item or style. Another style cop is the catty person who wants to feel herself the most stylish person around. If she knocks your style she can feel better about her own. There are

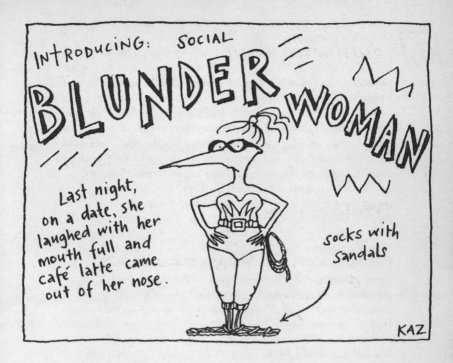

also fashion writers and freelance journalists filling up space around the ads in magazines and newspapers.

Come with me into the bossy-boots world of the style police. Carry a stout stick and don't be afraid to lay about yourself with it if you see any battalions of fashion writers whingeing about how our clothes look at least 17 minutes out of date. Come with me first into one of the most obvious areas of the style police: the wedding organisers. No! No! Oh, all right, I promise we won't be here long.

Oh my *lord:* have you ever seen so many rules in all your *life?* The dress has to be white. The dress has to be cream. The dress has to be elegant and simple. The dress has to be feminine and frilly. The dress has to look like a dangerous explosion in an organza factory during a cyclone. There must be expensive flowers. There must be an expensive photographer. You must have your facial three days before the wedding, your hair done, your nails done, your make-up done, blah, blah, and quite frankly, more blah. (And have you read our sensational *Blah Supplement?*)

The wedding dress is usually at the end of each high couture show, the most expensive item, the climax of the show, as in days gone past and in some quarters, a wedding is supposed to be the climax of a lifetime.

Take a closer look at that special supplement about the right way to get married. Look at all those advertisements around it and scattered through it. What a con. If you want to carry roses from your Aunty Lavinia's garden and get married in a nice old dress you found at the charity shop, you do it. The only ones screaming will be those you might have hired or bought from if you'd swallowed the 'rules', which were mostly made up by people who profit from them.

Fashion crime and fashion criminals

In the space-filling, get-somebody-else-to-do-most-of-the-thinking-for-this-article tradition of journalism (hey, I know about this, I've done it myself) comes the '50 all-time fashion disasters according to the experts' type story, and of course the snide 'worst dressed' lists and photographs with nasty captions in women's magazines. This kind of stuff makes us all into the style police. We can say, hey, that actor may have millions of dollars but she looks absolutely shocking in a puce velvet Heidi frock. It's the revenge of the ordinary against the (literally) well-heeled.

The opposite to this is the designers and clothes sellers telling us what's a fashion 'crime'. This is the revenge of the well-heeled on the ordinary – a chance for fashion designers to get really narky at us for not doing everything they tell us.

A leading Sunday paper, prompted by its panel of experts (almost all of them clothes manufacturers and sellers), says we can't wear body-hugging dresses if we 'don't have the right body to hug'. The wrong body, said the newspaper, has a 'protruding bottom and tummy'. Well, I do beg your pardon, but if your bottom doesn't protrude you've probably lost it entirely, in which case I suggest you contact a doctor.

Of course, this sort of thing is passed off as helpful hints, like the 'right' swimsuit to wear to 'camouflage' the body's 'defects'. Or, as

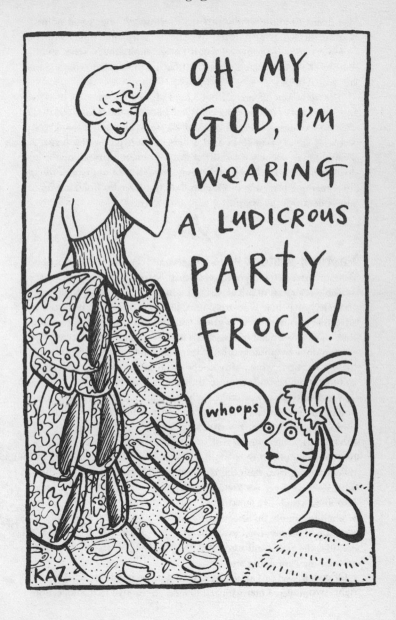

one magazine more kindly put it, 'to show off your good points'. Various drawings of women are shown with the 'right' and the 'wrong' swimsuit for her to wear. For example, the 'wrong' swimsuit for the 'pear-shaped' woman (that is, most adult women) has horizontal stripes.

The 'right' one apparently has a kind of a scarfy arrangement at the top, draped over the shoulders and tied between the breasts and three different colours on the rest of it with a stripe pointing down like an arrow at about waist level and a dark section below the waist. A swimsuit even vaguely resembling this has never been seen by me on any swimsuit racks. And I have been through a lot of them, looking for something plain and black that does not have leg holes cut up to just underneath the armpits.

Fashion writers

From a consumer's point of view, a good fashion writer will present new clothes, classics and a range of what's available at a range of prices, using photographs that show the clothes accurately on people who are shaped like the consumers. But from an advertiser's point of view, a good fashion writer runs glamorous pictures of its clothes and makes them look desirable and different. This is often done by photographing them in front of some children in a 'travel' location, which also keeps the tourism industry advertisers and the photo crew (including the fashion writer) happy as well.

We should be very careful of who is telling us what to wear on our bodies and on our faces. As photographer Bruce Weber says of the three writers he admires the most, 'What these women really have in common is that they're styling what their life is, what *their own* lives are about.' It's very scary when these women just might be insecure, neurotic, unhappy, too busy to consider the rights and wrongs of what they are doing and are subject to the whims of advertisers in their magazines.

— An English Fashion designer told me to wear high heels with jeans. Should I listen?
— No.

American writer Cynthia Heimel

A high-powered international fashion editor goes to the collections

156

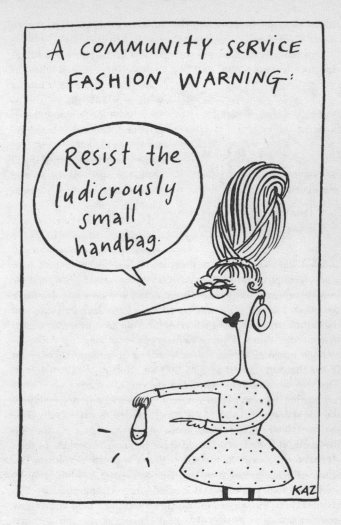

and private showings. She chooses some clothes. She organises a contra-deal, that is, a free trip to somewhere exotic if she can afford it in return for free 'plugs' in the magazine. Once there, she unpacks the clothes, the models, hopes the photographer won't get malaria, and gaffer tapes the back of the frocks to make them sit just right on the thin models. She tries to make the shoot 'interesting', perhaps even 'creative', or chooses a photographer with such ambitions.

Sometimes, she tells you in the text next to the photo that something's an 'essential'. This could be a white shirt, a ruched tulle skirt with velour tassels or a hairpin with a plastic daisy on it. Sometimes the fashion editor is desperate. But the fashion editor is never, ever, infallible. Sometimes she says stupid things about stupid clothes and changes her mind by autumn. That's her job.

> Keep a pair of high-heeled slippers in your bathroom.
>
> Britt Ekland
>
> Keep a hedgehog in your underpants – it would be more comfortable.
>
> Hermoine the Modern Girl

I was fashion writer at a newspaper for about three weeks. If it ever happens to you and you don't want to be a fashion editor, here's what you do. Run a story with pictures of a Paris designer's coat (about £500) and the local department store's coat (about £300) and how you can make one yourself (about £30), and wait for the Paris designer's shop and the department store, a big advertiser in your newspaper, to scream blue murder. You will not be fashion editor for long.

Vogue magazine is regarded as an arbiter of fashion. At last count it was charging more than £11,000 for a full-page advertisement. That's 11 thousand reasons not to upset the advertisers.

Longtime icon and *Vogue* editor Diana Vreeland once (although she was at *Harper's Bazaar* at the time) decided to write a new fashion law. 'We're going to eliminate all handbags', she announced, explaining that designers would have to provide pockets in their clothes for women. At the time, this was pretty revolutionary. Someone was summoned to Vreeland to explain how things really worked. 'I think you've lost your mind,' she said diplomatically. 'Do you realise our income from handbag advertising is God knows how many millions a year?' Exactly. And *Harper's Bazaar* did not then announce the death of the handbag.

chapter *five*

Hyper hype

Lotions and potions

Big bucks First, we pause for a small mind boggle. Wholesale sales of cosmetics and toiletries are more than £2.25 billion a year in Britain. Thirteen per cent of this is in moisturisers and cleansers. Worldwide, the cosmetics industry is worth £10 billion a year, with normal profit margins of more than 50 per cent.

Moisturisers and anti-wrinkle creams The Dermatologists (skin specialists) say a good moisturiser will temporarily smooth and 'plump' out wrinkles only because it is adding water to the skin. This plumping-out effect makes no lasting change to skin, all of which, no matter what you slather on, is always getting older.

Asked whether expensive creams are better, they offer this cost-benefit analysis. 'You might get a 90 per cent improvement with aqueous cream and a 95 per cent improvement with something that costs 10 or 20 times as much.' That 5 per cent difference is probably not visible with the naked eye. Only 5 to 10 per cent of people have a naturally dry skin and really 'need' a moisturiser.

In 1986 *Choice* magazine had 800 people use 90 over-the-counter

159

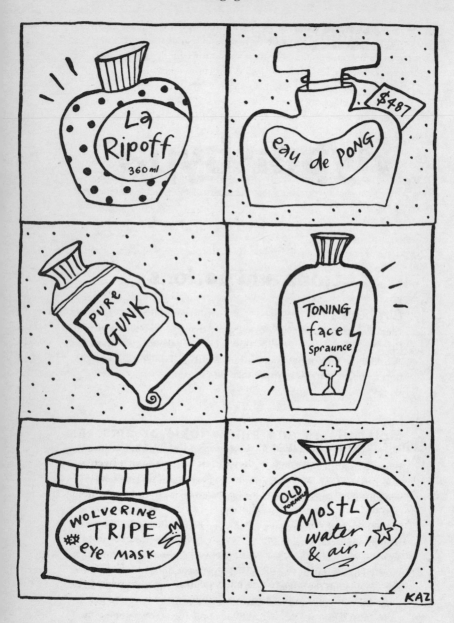

moisturisers given to them in unlabelled bottles. Plain, cheap chemists' aqueous cream, made from vaseline, glycerine and water, rated as high or higher than the expensive stuff with designer names. (It can be watered down if you find it not runny enough.)

If you're a young woman, you probably won't care much about moisturisers until you're in your late twenties. The simple truth is that a sunhat might save you thousands of dollars in creams and lotions. Especially if you don't drink heavily or smoke.

Dermatologists estimate that about 80 per cent of what used to be thought normal ageing of the skin is actually 'photo-ageing', due to exposure to sunlight. We are spending millions trying to correct it with creams and treatments that are scientifically unable to repair the damage.

Which? Way to Health magazine carried out a survey on anti-ageing moisturisers. They asked six manufacturers for evidence to back up the claims made for their products. Nothing. Six months later they asked again, and three companies provided information – too late to go to press. A panel of dermatologists who also checked out the creams was not impressed by the anti-ageing claims made for the products. They pronounced them, on the whole, moisturisers with sunscreen. So don't be taken in by expensive lotions with fancy packaging and extravagant claims. It's all just fat, dahlings.

This has to be balanced against sensible precautions and living a full life not locked away inside thinking what a nice skin you've got. But if you're actually sunbaking, looking for a tan, you're looking for trouble.

What is a moisturiser? Moisturisers are either humectants, which add water to sit on top of the skin, or fats that form a layer, making it harder for water in the skin to 'evaporate' in air-conditioning or other drying environments. Either way, it's not particularly complicated. It's a case of 'just add water' – you choose how much, which way and the cost.

Dermatologists insist that the newer, extra ingredients in moisturisers, such as collagen and elastin, cannot be absorbed into the skin, despite the claims of cosmetic companies. Even Unilever's own chemist said collagen didn't do much of anything when rubbed into the top layer of skin. It's a molecule thing – like trying to get a yak through the hole in your letterbox.

Placentas – animal and, some say, human – were big for a while as ingredients. Hyaluronic acid, introduced in the 1980s, is claimed to 'deliver' more water to the skin. Then came 'lipids' (just fats) and 'liposomes', supposed to deliver ingredients below the upper surface of the epidermis (skin) but not necessarily do anything after they arrived (sort of like dull house guests).

Liposomes, weeny molecules, are the 'taxis' used to deliver fancy ingredients below the surface of the skin. This allows moisturiser ads to use diagrams with arrows showing the moisturiser 'getting into' the skin. But even liposome 'taxis' will only take the moisturiser halfway. So far, no product can be delivered to the dermis where the body makes its own collagen and elastin. And even if such a long-distance 'taxi' were to be invented, there's no evidence that any added moisturiser at the dermis level would do anything except arrive.

Despite the fact that dermatologists and even the manufacturers of many cosmetics insist that after billions of dollars of research over decades not one – *not one* – potion has been invented that will interfere in any way with the ageing process, *New Idea* magazine chose to run an article on cosmetic ingredients, headed 'Anti-ageing breakthroughs'.

If a cosmetic company itself had made that claim it could have been reported to Trading Standards for misleading advertising, unless it proved on reasonable grounds that a cream reversed or stopped the ageing process. *New Idea* ran the phone numbers of 13 cosmetics companies corresponding with products mentioned in the article. With friends like these you can reduce your advertising budget. But the magazine can't have been too sure about when to report a 'breakthrough' – the article was published 18 months after it was written. The truth is that cosmetics companies announce 'breakthroughs' on a regular basis as an advertising tool.

Buzzwords Ceramides A fat. Putting fat on the skin does not change the skin any more than peanut butter on a sandwich alters the state of the bread. *New Idea* still called ceramides 'another breakthrough miracle ingredient'.

Hyaluronic acid Made from roosters' combs. Dermatologists are sceptical of its ability to be absorbed properly once it is delivered to the epidermis. One likened the acid molecule to a length of piano wire and the skin to a bucket of water.

Liposomes These are fatty droplets extracted from eggs or from 'plant extracts'. But basically they're fat. One magazine called them 'tiny, round, leakproof packages made of skin-friendly lipids'. Oh, *cute*. Lipids are of course just fats. Dermatologists agree that liposomes only penetrate the upper skin. Some sellers of liposome products say that the product alters cells in the upper skin, but research from Christian Dior was not performed on human skin but cells from mice spleens. (I don't know about you, but if there's one thing I can't stand it's a wrinkly mouse spleen.)

Elastin/Collagen Normal skin at the dermis level contains elastin and collagen, which are damaged and altered by sunlight, possibly by UVB rays which are only stopped by opaque creams, clothing or a solid hat. Added collagens and elastins usually come from animal fats and tissue. According to a Health Department spokesperson, 'stuff like elastin has simply ginormous molecules. They simply can't get in'.

Retin-A Retin-A (tretinoin cream based on retinoic acid, a vitamin A derivative) was developed as an acne cream and in the UK is available only on prescription. In Australia, however, it was also sold in tens of millions of tubes over the counter as a new, amazing face-peeling wrinkle treatment. Other creams were also marketed with retinoic or tretinoic acid. More than one magazine called Retin-A a 'miracle cream'.

The *Lancet* medical journal ran an article on the link between the use of vitamin-A derivative therapeutic creams during pregnancy and birth defects. Although manufacturers of the creams insist that no link has been proven, the general recommendation is that Retin-A not be used in pregnancy or when pregnancy is likely.

Retin-A damages the skin of some users, causing it to become red and inflamed and come off in flakes. This side-effect 'generally settles down' during or after use, according to dermatologists.

Retin-A and its colleague products are, so far, the only truly 'therapeutic' treatments available. 'Therapeutic' doesn't mean it's necessarily good, it means that the product has been shown to change the body. Retin-A was registered as a therapeutic good because of its effect on acne.

Acid trips Alpha Hydroxy Acids (AHAs) are found naturally in plants (often fruit) and dairy products. And now they're in cosmetics. They're another 'miracle' being advertised. The acid is supposed to loosen the 'glue' that binds dead cells to the skin's surface to reveal a fresher, new layer underneath.

When Estée Lauder launched a fruit-acid cream called Fruition in the US, with much more extravagant claims than those made previously for fruit-acid products – 'up to 18 per cent reduction in the appearance of fine lines and wrinkles' and '60 per cent increase in skin clarity' – it captured 10 per cent of skin care sales within weeks. Think about that 18 per cent. Could you tell if a wrinkle looked less than 20 per cent deeper?

Dermatologists point out that acid skin peels are done with very powerful acids that shouldn't be used unless under the care of a skin doctor. The glycolic acid used in a skin peel stings and burns when applied and is left for up to five minutes.

Even dermatologists admit that fruit acids cannot cure wrinkles, only diminish them in some cases over a period of time. And considering that wrinkles stay in the same place while top layers come and go, nothing is really being changed by just stripping the layers off earlier than they would usually go naturally.

Deeper peels can take up to a week to heal. Personally, I can't see how this can be a sensible thing to do to the skin. This is how that whole *Phantom of the Opera* thing started, isn't it? People running around chucking acid on other people's faces?

A too-potent skin peel causes severe blistering, scarring and a whitening or darkening of the skin. This nasty attack on the skin, this peeling and scraping and scrubbing is kind of weird and over the top. Naomi Wolf pointed out in *The Beauty Myth* that Clinique says, 'Do it as aggressively as possible'. But leave some steel wool for the dishes?

Again women are supposed to submit to pain as some kind of duty.

Secret advertising A dermatologist explains the scam simply. 'Week after week manufacturers' claims, accompanied by glossy photographs, land on the desks of beauty editors around the world. These heavily biased, subjective blurbs, with the photographs captioned, then appear unedited in the magazines as virtually unpaid advertisements masquerading as independent editorial copy.' This is cheap for the magazine and even cheaper for the companies. The only losers are those of us who expect a more critical analysis and those who believe everything they read. Once you know how the scam works, you can cast a much more critical eye over the 'new products' columns, the beauty stories, the make-overs, and your local newspaper's ads for beauty salons and weight treatments as well.

General fibbing One reason why flashy moisturisers cost 20 times as much as aqueous cream is not the expensive ingredients but the amount spent in advertising that the company has to make back in sales.

You know the paid, glossy cosmetics advertisements, usually the most expensive full-page, right-hand-side ads in the women's magazines? And the prime time TV ads? Dermatologists are especially concerned that the advertisements suggest that 'damage' – from the sun or ageing – can be reversed. This is a lie.

In the US, several companies have been fined over faffing on fallaciously (that's fibbing) about what their products could do. Effeto Immediato Spa Lift for Face, manufacturer Princess Marcella Borghese claimed, was 'formulated with the revolutionary "Involctin

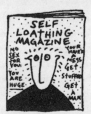

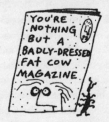

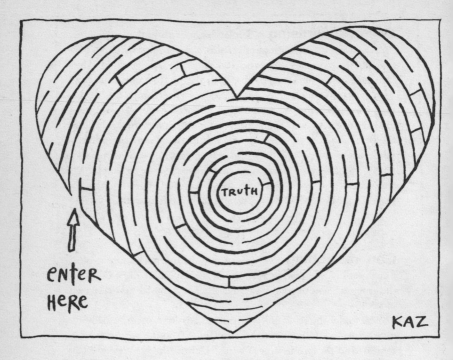

Protein Complex" and the Aqua de Vita "Living Water" Complex (and) it works to replace skin's natural source of firmness'. *Ms* magazine revealed that the only active ingredient in the $40 bottle was sunscreen.

In Europe, too, companies should be told to pull their heads in.

Legal lies Essentially, cosmetics ads can get away with lying about what the creams can do, but not about what's *in* the product. In 1990, a spokesman for the Australian Trade Practices Commission put it this way: 'They can say you'll be radiantly lovely and men will goggle at you if you use their products but if they say they contain crushed iguana nostrils they had better contain crushed iguana nostrils.' I read this quote back to a spokeswoman for the Commission in 1993 and she agreed.

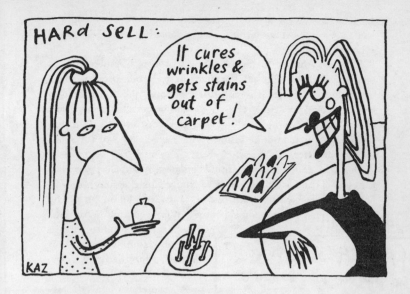

In the UK Trading Standards can prosecute a company for misleading or deceptive advertising claims. They may investigate outrageous claims such as 'slows the ageing process', but only on complaint. The 'dispute' is considered to be between the complainant and the manufacturer. One little person and one great big, rich company.

Science fibbing Sometimes it seems you need a degree in scientific language to translate some of these ads. But apparently, this is actually a handicap.

According to dermatologists, none of this stuff works. The ads are deliberately pseudo-scientific, and the more you know about science the harder it is to make out what they're saying.

Nivea asks, 'Isn't technology beautiful?' and says its double layer liposomes (fats, remember) deliver 'precious moisture'. The 'Ponds Institute' in the TV ads is staffed by languid women in white coats. Clinique is proud of its skin analysis 'computer', which is really just a dinky wee plastic thingy with knobs on it. Check one out on a cosmetics counter at a department store near you. They might as well do you a drawing on the back of a paper bag with a stubby old eyebrow pencil.

Elizabeth Arden's 'Ceramide Time Complex Capsules...Phenomenon' is pictured like a flying saucer in space, quite near Neptune by the look of things. It is said that this boosts the skin hydration level up to 450 per cent after an hour (and wastes a lot of individual plastic in the capsules). That 450 per cent, while sounding humungous, would not be visible to the naked eye so you couldn't tell the difference.

Dior's Svelte is a 'new scientific conquest by the Christian Dior laboratories', and is claimed to have 'anti-cellulite activity...the silhouette [is] liberated and transformed...a true revolution, proven by tests performed under medical control'. Whose control? What tests?

Has my silhouette been detained somewhere? Does Amnesty International know about this?

A cosmetics counter saleswoman shows customers a 'diagram' of a 'plant extract liposome' being swallowed by a skin cell. The Australasian College of Dermatologists says this is impossible. Fat molecules and collagen molecules cannot *enter* cells. They're way too big. Try to imagine getting your kitchen table down the sink plughole and you'll get the picture.

French fibbing My favourite cosmetics ads are the ones that faff on in French. Even the exported goods only for overseas sales from France have the names in French still on them. In the *Addams Family* television show and movies, when Morticia speaks French her husband Gomez swoons with desire and starts kissing her arms. French names in advertising are supposed to have a similar effect on us.

Why say 'concentrated gel' when you can say 'Gel Con-centré Multi-Actif'? Doesn't 'Eclat de Jeunesse' sound less unlikely than 'Burst of youth'? And 'Buste Galbe et Fermeté' more sophisticated than 'Bust shape and firmness'? You can get respect, serenity, balance and curves in a bottle and it sounds more plausible in French – *respectée, serenissime, harmonie* and *galbeor*. What a load of *merde*.

Environmental hazards At a recent seminar on women's health and the environment in North America, the conference was told that seemingly unrelated problems, from cancer to menstrual disorders, infertility and chronic fatigue syndrome, often resulted from women's unique susceptibility to environmental poisons such as pesticides and lead.

It was reported that the essential female hormone oestrogen is vulnerable to such poisoning. Breast cancer has been linked to a higher concentration of DDT pesticides and other organochlorins in the blood. Women in the petroleum and chemical industries have a higher rate of breast cancer.

In the face of a poisoned earth, all the cosmetics companies suggest to tackle the problem is spreading more fat on your face.

Estée Lauder claims that its Advanced Night Repair Protective Recovery Complex will 'help prevent environmental damage: ultraviolet rays and free radicals'. Free radicals are unstable molecules – feral sciencey things that the skin produces when it is exposed to sunlight or pollution. Free radicals run amok and break down the elasticity of the skin.

Clarins' Power Moisturiser claims 'the power of environmental protection. Safeguard skin's beauty from the visible effects of environmental aggression and air pollution.' Monteil's Ice Monteil moisturiser 'intercepts skin-damaging "toxic hazards" before ageing effects begin to show'. Odelys promised to help with 'stress, pollution and the hectic pace of modern living' with plant and marine extracts.

Bioelements has a product called Urban Detox. *Elle* magazine claimed on its behalf that 'it protects skin from dangerous environmental hazards while it neutralises the formation of free radicals that lead to premature ageing'.

If we continue to give more priority to our skin care than to our planet care, we're going to have a worse environment and worse skin, because it absolutely can't be fixed once it's damaged (that's the skin, not the planet).

The brainy briny 'Marine technologies', which usually turns out to mean seaweed or plankton, mud (it's called *fange* in France, chérie) or just plain old sea water, are other miracle cosmetic ingredients that pop up now and then. *Diet and Lifestyle* magazine practically wet itself about sea water. 'It's naturally alive, containing living organisms, which have a self-purifying and rejuvenating power.' Not to mention anchovies, squid and in selected world locations, oil spills. All this may make you feel good, but again, there's no evidence of skin penetration benefits.

This didn't stop *Mademoiselle* magazine from faffing, 'According to our skin-care forecast, a new wave of seaweed-based products may help fight acne, fend off wrinkles, even block sun damage.' The sources for the story included the president and founder of a company selling the first seaweed-based skin-care line in the US, a vice-president of research and development at Estée Lauder and (ha, now we're getting somewhere!) a vice-president of 'creative marketing' for Revlon.

Cleansers Plain, unscented soap and water will do – honest. Cosmetics industry research shows that their fancy claims about special cleansing lotions have been ignored by the 70 per cent of women who still use soap and water to clean their faces. Accordingly, the companies now flog soaps that make the same claims as the lotions. Or they say you need special moisturising to counter the drying effect of the soap. (Only unusually dry skins should not be washed with soap.)

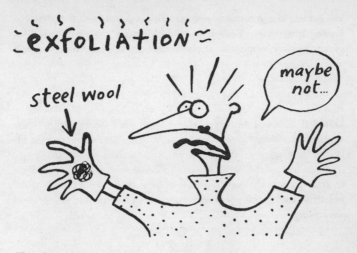

Toning Guess what? Toners are completely unnecessary, a con. Most toners contain alcohol and, like aftershaves, they are supposed to constrict the pores after cleansing and before moisturising. 'Toning is basically a waste of time and money. The products...basically consist of water, alcohol and glycerine,' sums up one dermatologist. The only thing a toner might usefully do is help remove detergents from washing with soap but a good rinse with water does that too. All a toner will do is make you feel pampered. What toners do very well is look pretty-pretty in their artificial colours of pink and blue, often in sexy, curvaceous designer bottles (a lot more curvaceous than they say we should be).

Exfoliation This means sloughing off dead skin cells, speeding up a natural process. Various scrubs are available. A gentle face washer with soap and water will do a lot of it. Companies will try and sell you volcanic mud, apricot seeds and everything else short of driveway gravel for the job.

Hypo-allergenic cosmetics This means designed for sen-

171

sitive skins, so not carrying extra fragrances or colours. Some people confuse it with 'hyper-allergenic', thinking it is likely to cause allergic reactions. A hypo-allergenic product doesn't guarantee you will not be allergic to it.

Drugs 'Cosmeceuticals' is the clumsy word being suggested to explain the blurred crossover between drugs and cosmetics. Acids fall into this category because they change the structure and/or function of a part of the body. Cosmetics companies are not registering these as drugs and some say this is because they would then be subject to greater scrutiny and regulation about testing, distribution and advertising.

Safety labelling The long-term effects of many products are simply unknown and although in the USA cosmetics must be labelled with a full list of ingredients, in the UK we will have to wait until 1997, when an EC directive leaps into action. The label must include a list of all ingredients (but not the quantities), so people can check for anything they're allergic to. Pamphlets must be available at point of sale for items too small for a label, such as lipstick. But according to one chemist, 'That doesn't help you or me very much because you need a degree in organic chemistry to understand what the compounds are.'

On average, a lipstick wearer will swallow 4.5 kilos of lipstick over 40 years, says Professor Geoffrey Duggin, head of toxicology at the Royal Prince Alfred Hospital, New South Wales. He worries that of more than 10,000 chemicals used in cosmetics, only about 500 have been tested. 'For too long people have assumed that cosmetics are harmless and that they simply sit on the skin. We now know that a lot of people absorb a lot of drugs through their skin.'

Although allergic reactions are rare, consumers do need the detailed labelling to protect themselves.

real *gorgeous*

Nature and nurture Some newer companies are producing 'natural' cosmetics. These products have feel-good smell-good components such as essential oils, non-animal soaps, vegetable and plant extracts. Many also have chemical preservatives. Some herbal products are very expensive for no obvious reason, and some people are allergic to natural substances.

Most of the 'natural' products avoid animal extracts, which means (don't read on if you're a queasy type) you miss out on ambergris (from whales) and dried beaver's genitals in perfumes; collagen (animal tissue) and hyaluronic acid (from roosters' combs) in moisturisers; oestrogen (from pregnant horse's wee); tallow (animal fat) in soap, lipstick, and shampoos, and spermaceti (more poor whaley bits) in creams and shampoos. Sometimes these will be given alternative scientific names to further disguise their ancestry.

Clarins advertises geranium, ivy, aloe, lavender, mint and many more yummy-sounding things without saying exactly what they are supposed to do apart from being 'natural'. The 'skin firming concentrate' has horsetail, horse chestnut, pineapple and condurango, which I previously had pegged as a Peruvian dissident's club. Egg white and gelatine are also used in many moisturisers because they tighten the skin until they are washed off again.

Did you ever imagine something called hyaluronic acid was from roosters' combs? I guess 'New improved dead chook bits in a can!' doesn't quite have the same allure.

Further information

Your local chemist will tell you about cheap aqueous cream.

Make-up

Going without vs getting slathered All the women we have presented to us as role models are wearing make-up – in magazines, in films, on television. A large proportion of the make-up

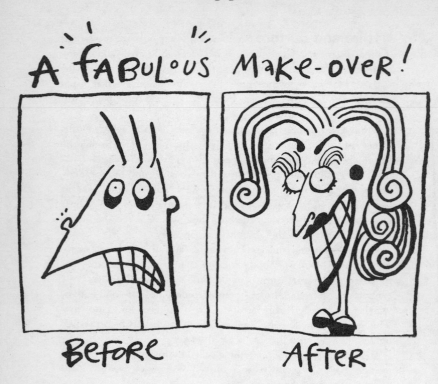

industry is even structured around buying expensive make-up which will not look like make-up – an artifice to cover blemishes and variations, and the perverse 'natural'-coloured lipstick.

We are told that without make-up we look tired, washed out, we are not making the effort; we feel, even, that we 'haven't got our face on'. Women are not supposed to look tired or strung out or sick or in trouble. All things that show up in a face and can be masked by make-up. These real emotions and afflictions must be hidden and unacknowledged. We must pretend. Put on a happy face.

Don't expect magazines to tell you that your face is better off breathing without make-up, or that the no-make-up look is perfectly fine. Their advertisers would have a *fit*. Or possibly kittens.

The make-up sellers and the magazines in their thrall have done very well in turning around the public image of make-up. Before the 1920s, a woman openly wearing make-up was likely to be

174

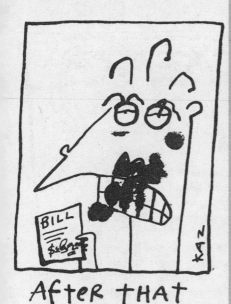

After that

> I still remember a day a week
> into my first office job when I
> came into work without foun-
> dation on. My dress was neat
> and clean, my hair tidy and I
> felt presentable in an office. I
> was told by my boss that I was
> not to come into the office
> without make-up on. I remem-
> ber feeling insulted and that
> my face without make-up was
> my personal choice, but of
> course being young and inex-
> perienced agreed to the
> request. I don't any more.
> What made the situation worse
> as far as I'm concerned is that
> my boss was a female.
>
> Delys, 24

shunned from 'polite' society as a strumpet (what a great word).

When you're just becoming a teenager, the world of teenage magazines seems glamorous and mysterious. I learned from them that
you couldn't just do nothing to yourself. I learned that there was, in
fact, an exhaustive amount of stuff you had to do to be a teenage girl.
Boys could just throw on a T-shirt and walk out the door (although
I'm sure a lot of them did air-guitar and hair smoothing and checking for whiskers in front of the mirror) but we had work to do and
a lot more products to spend money on. We had to transform ourselves into somebody else. We not only had to 'make the effort'. We
had to be seen to make the effort.

Ask anyone who has come out the other side of adolescence if
they'd go back and do it again and the only takers would be deeply
insane. It's a time of vulnerability, change, groping around for an
identity and a sexuality. At a deeply impressionable time, when all

you want to do is be over it and be an adult, one of the lessons of how to be an adult that girls learn is to wear make-up. At a time of being at best radiantly crabby, the messages tell us that if we looked better, we'd feel better.

Even a little girl learns by watching the world around her that putting on make-up is what grown-up women do. When she plays dress-ups she puts on some lipstick and clomps around in some high-heeled shoes that are too big for her. This is what she first is taught about what it is to be a woman. And she has learned it from observing us.

Make-up can be heaps of fun but it's not compulsory.

Essentially confused 'What could be worse than finding you've left your make-up bag at home?' asks a *Fashion Quarterly* hack, who has obviously never been held up at the letterbox by three rabid Rottweilers and an ex-boyfriend asking for a £1000 loan.

The article continues, 'Suddenly that nondescript but morale-boosting bag of powders and creams seems to hold the key to your true identity. In fact, it's hard to imagine how you will get through the day without it. Every woman totes around a make-up bag of essential items to cover any kind of emergency, from simple retouch jobs to a complete overhaul after a workout at the gym. For most people, a blusher is essential...' and on and on it goes.

This is often the problem with beauty editors and writers. Because of the world they live in, they get convinced of a few things. You can't be beautiful without 'product' unless you're a supermodel. Your identity is in a bag. An eyebrow brush is essential. Ha. They actually seem unaware that many women never use blusher; that some use it only at night for big events; that some of us carry only a lipstick on a night out and nothing at all during the day. They have bought the hype from the companies that buy advertising to pay their salaries.

Part of the hype suggests that there is no natural beauty without minimalist make-up foundation and translucent powder and 'nude' lipstick and tortured eyebrows. The sections called 'beauty' are about selling. The word 'beauty' has been, um, slightly hijacked. It's all a bit

> I didn't know how to talk to males. I would pack on the make-up to try and make an impression – make-up for me was also a face to hide behind. I started to make male friends and now talk to most as I would a female friend. And for the record I wear very little make-up now – and my skin is benefiting from the change! It would take me up to one and a half hours to get ready of a morning. It now takes me less than half the time.
>
> Sandy, 19

confusing in the magazines, really, when dangerous diet suggestions might be found under 'health' and boxing as a good exercise idea under 'beauty'.

Beauty pages You know the beauty pages in glossy magazines? Where they run photos of new products and a little paragraph on each one? This is not because the beauty editors have been scouring the shops, getting products independently tested and deciding which ones are the best to recommend. It's because press releases and free samples arrive at the office all day long. And very often, the paragraph about the product is just exactly word for word what the manufacturer says about it in the press release.

There is no questioning of the claims, no matter how confusing. 'Guerlain's Protective Base for the Eyelids is like a mini-foundation and powder-in-one for the eye area, allowing make-up to slide on more easily, and fixing it in place.' Say what?

Or 'These three colours are set to become classics. Sold as singles, they also blend together brilliantly,' says a beauty page about pink, brown and blue eyeshadows. Blend blue and pink for purple and that losing boxer look! Or blend blue and brown for that kind of muddy, erky look!

And the beauty page is often dominated by a misleading photograph of a model from the magazine's files who isn't wearing one single scrap of any of the make-up on the page. Or it might be a photograph supplied by the make-up company. Either way it has been professionally lit, photographed and made-up.

And now magazines are crediting the *perfume* the model is supposedly wearing. In a photograph. What next? 'And Juniper is also

177

wearing a Lil-lets.' Anyway, beauty pages are not critical (in the true sense of the word), or analytical, or questioning, or, most often, anything but unpaid ads.

So too are the 'make-over' stories: often with similar cheating on what products are actually used and how exclusively. And the 'new beauty looks' articles, with pretend history lessons like, 'Not since the 1950s has eyeliner been so important', and recommendation of what colours are in fashion. The 'after' photographs are usually better lit with the guinea pig smiling.

And guess what? It's not all on the beauty pages either but escaped and running amok through the rest of the magazine. When the atrocious *Hair, Body and Beauty* magazine ran a story called 'beauty hints for flirts' it mentioned no fewer than 27 specific products, not to mention suggesting that you practise flirting with your father. (Oh pur-*lease*.)

Lollies What *is* irresistible about the beauty pages is the way they mash up the lipsticks and shake out the coloured powders and scribble with the lip-liners and squish the eye paint around. Doesn't it all look scrumptious? I love this part. I think because I just love paints and crayons and gorgeous colours. I'm not sure it would look so attractive if it were not spilled artistically over a glowing light box but all over my bathroom instead. Then it would be an over-priced mess.

> Wearing make-up is asking for approval. Wearing make-up is an apology for our actual faces. Wearing make-up makes it seem as if a woman has something to hide. Wearing make-up makes a woman look older than she actually is.
>
> American writer Cynthia Heimel

But ahhhh, in the magazines! All art-directed and enticing! It's like a whole lot of glorious lollies. Good enough to eat but pretty enough just to look at in those pretty jars, or all right, I admit it, smushed all over the light box.

Despite the fact that *Glamour* magazine make-up survey results of April 1993 showed that women want *less* packaging in cosmetics (as well as better sales help, more samples, privacy at the counter, sunscreens and no animal testing), we often choose for the look of a

---

---

range. Some women put their plain aqueous cream into designer bottles, sneaky old possums.

Trends Ignore all trends in make-up. Otherwise you would be a true fashion victim with a pastel look and false eyelashes one minute, the minimalist (strangely expensive) look the next and then the full-on accident in a blusher factory caricature. You'll be spending £20 on a 'Chanel Brilliant Soleil Sheer Lipstick'. That's £20 for the no-lipstick look! You could get the same effect with Vaseline, one suspects. Or buying waterproof mascara which is rarely anything like waterproof; sometimes it's barely blinkproof. (And beware of mascara without enough preservative in it or old mascara you find under the car seat or in the cutlery drawer. The resultant bacteria can cause permanent eye damage.) Find what you like and experiment without costing yourself a fortune.

The snake pit Rather than rush out and buy all the stuff, take a trip to the nearest mall and try on the testers – being very careful about allergies and transferred germs, of course. This can be fun. But remember the women behind the counter are aliens. They are robots at the front line of the most cut-throat high mark-up phenomenal profit business there is.

The cosmetics and perfume counters in department stores are known in the trade as the snake pit. These women will lie, insult

> *Magazine editor at meeting to decide what is going in a women's magazine:* 'Right, beauty, and make it quick.'
> *Beauty editor:* 'Clarins, Shiseido, Paloma Picasso, Chanel, make-up, Germolene, lipsticks, powder bases, faces, eyes, lips, nostrils. This is all off the top of my head. Douching with mint is a thought. Ten tips for tropical toenails. I'm thinking natural zing. Moist is my word de jour. Skin is in. Lovely wet, moist lips. Wet droplets. Sun, sea, sand, water, waves, beach. I see a photo shoot. I'm looking at two weeks in the Caribbean. And the usual – try and be more beautiful if you want to have more sex.'
>
> From *Absolutely Fabulous* by Jennifer Saunders

you gently, undermine your confidence and put disquieting names to problems you never knew you had because they're not problems. Be careful that instead of letting you play with the paints for fun, they don't turn you into a quivering mass of melting self-esteem, obsessed with pore size (it's genetic and NOTHING sold changes it), eyebrow shape, lip-liner and the like.

Some of those women work on a commission so they get more money for everything they convince you to buy. Others, of course, are darlings and will whisper that you can get a cheaper version at the counter over there which actually works better. Or they will *trick* you by being nice and saying you have lovely skin you don't need any of these but your eyes might as well be in Poland for all I can see of them, try this divine mascara and let me just cover up your whole face and obliterate your whole identity now hold still or else.

Make a pact with a friend that you will each buy only one thing after testing lots of them and make each other stick to it. Don't forget that you're mostly paying for packaging, which accounts for 60 per cent of the price and the advertising, as well as the salary of this woman standing there trying to look like your skin is the most tragic thing since the invasion of Panama. Or they'll make you 'over' and tell you that orange tones are absolutely adorable on you. This is bound to be a filthy lie.

It's always harder for you girls in the country but think of all the money you're saving. And don't forget that while city girls are paying for the expensive big-name brands, your closest chemist sells the same stuff, the same shades, only cheaper in different packaging.

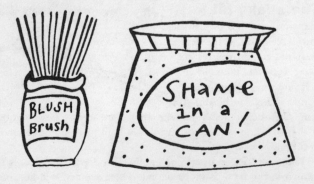

Avoid those bulk mail orders of lots of cosmetics: why let somebody else choose for you?

Blusher Before Elizabeth Arden Coral Coquette Luxury Cheek Colour and its other modern counterparts, women would pinch their cheeks to bring colour into them. You may be naturally pale, or you may not be getting enough good food for a naturally rosy glow. Most blusher looks fake, unless it's lit and photographed by a professional.

Anyway, the real thing is so awful — I mean blushing. You know, going red and then everyone notices and you can't stop going red, and I'm going red just writing this remembering the other times I've gone red and even my ears went red and the times I've gone red and I haven't even been embarrassed I've been furious or confused or embarrassed for somebody else. Aaaaarrgghhhh! It's feeling, as one friend says, like a caged beetroot.

And yet here we are buying this product called blusher. It's a hangover from 'blushing bride' and other old fashioned notions of girls kept in the dark about sexual or important matters and 'blushing prettily' to show their innocence and girlhood. Bleuuugh.

Eyes Although there is virtually no regulation of the cosmetics industry in the US, the Food and Drug Administration there has warned against the use of eyebrow and eyelash dyes, saying 'there is

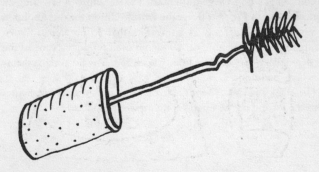

a risk of severe eye injury and even blindness'. Even vegetable dyes can cause allergic reactions.

A letter to a problem page I read in a waiting room had a sad letter from a woman who had gone one step further and had her eyebrows tattooed blue-black. One was higher than the other one, and a different shade, giving her a very bizarre permanent expression she couldn't do much about.

Don't buy the mascaras with extra filaments or bits to 'extend' or 'add to' lashes. You might end up trying to fish them out of your eyes all day. And what exactly is the point of the 'no colour' mascara? You might as well just comb your own eyelashes.

Animal testing
Companies that claim to have eliminated animal testing themselves can't guarantee that the chemicals they buy have not already been tested on animals.

The phrase 'cruelty-free' or 'not tested on animals' may mean only that the end product was not tested although each ingredient was.

Some companies use no new ingredients, choosing instead only from a 1978 European Economic Community list of proven safe ingredients. This means these companies cannot advertise amazing new breakthroughs or gobsmackingly sudden age-thwarting inventions. The herbal company Blackmores only uses ingredients that have not been tested on animals since 1985 when their safety was established. The Body Shop's cut-off point is 1989.

If you want to be as sure as possible that your cosmetics are made by companies who have genuinely tried to minimise their testing on animals, you can get a list from the British Union for the Abolition of Vivisection, which lists all companies that do no animal testing during the development of or on the finished product. None of the big department store counter brands are listed. The list also has shampoos and conditioners.

The other way to avoid animal testing is to stick with old favourites from the list and not be lured by the newer products.

Good enough to eat
Make-up colours are often named after foods. Forbidden to enjoy eating, women can have guilt-free Raisin (Clinique lip pencil), Rose Chocolat (Lancôme lippy), Cherries in the Snow (Revlon lippy) and a heap of caffeine kickstarters such as Mocha Dream and Cafe Au Lait.

A poll of *Mademoiselle* magazine staff and their favourite cosmetics produced a clear bias in favour of food names. One US company is kicking against the trend with names like 'Road-Kill', but it won't catch on. Leatrice Eiseman, of the avoidable-sounding Eiseman Centre of Color Information and Training in the US, says, 'A woman is more likely to buy and stay loyal to a Claret Red for example, than she is to a Number 12.'

Lipstick
Lipstick is the most common single cosmetic purchase. Most lipsticks are weighted to make it seem as if we're getting more for our money.

Hold just the lid of a lipstick in the palm of your hand and feel how light it is. Now feel the heavier base. The lipstick itself is very light, so you're paying for that extra weighting and packaging. The matt lipsticks have stronger colour. The gloss lipsticks are less drying. There are names like All Day Torrid Perfect Lipstick and New Geranium Luxury Lipstick, Golden Raisin Different Lipstick (pardon?), Café Chic Luxury Lipstick and even Anger. I am waiting for one called Torrid Crabby Luxurious Sultana Restaurant.

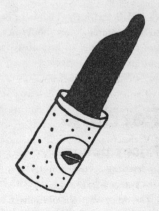

Further information

A full list of preferred products is available from: British Union for the Abolition of Vivisection, 16A Crane Grove, London N7 8LB. Phone 0171 700 4888. Some of the better-known preferred product make-up brands include Beauty Without Cruelty, the Body Shop and East of Eden. Many other companies are approved for other skin lotions, toothpastes, soaps, cleaning products, sunscreens, pet stuff and hair products.

The Vegan Society produce *The Animal-Free Shopper*, which provides information on where to buy vegan-friendly products. Contact them at: The Vegan Society, Donald Watson House, 7 Battle Road, St Leonards-on-Sea, East Sussex TN37 7AA. Phone 01424 427393.

Beauty Salons

A little luxury These are little offices we go to when we want to be pampered. They should not be torture chambers and we should not be expected to be transformed by them. For that we need a pumpkin and some mice.

Perfume

Pricey pongs The first known perfume factory was run by priests in sixteenth century Italy to help Europeans cover up the fact that personal hygiene had yet to be discovered. Back then, most people never washed themselves. (I'm sorry. These are facts. No wonder they all got Black Plague. Probably Black Plaque as well.) By 1900, bathing was more common. But more like once a week for the 'civilised' world (England, if you don't mind).

Queen Elizabeth I, after all, had announced that she had a bath once a month 'whether she needed it or not', and the eleventh Duke of Norfolk only ever had a wash when he got so drunk he passed out, whereupon the poor servants would give him a right going over with a scrubbing brush.

Perfumes in the early part of the twentieth century were considered only for 'fast' girls, which is to say girls who like to have a good time. Having a good time and admitting to liking it was considered MOST unladylike. But the first deodorant did not go on sale until the 1920s, so the richer, crabbier women decided that eau de Cologne, a watered-down version of perfume and the forerunner of 4711, which had been around since the 1700s, was acceptable.

Essential oils are now popular, marketed as cruelty-free, without musk (from deer glands), ambergris (bits of endangered whale) or chemicals. Like any other compound essential oils can cause allergic reactions. They can be used in burners, or on light globes to make a room or house fragrant, rather than a person. Many home-produced body lotions and bubble baths sold in boutiques and at markets are now being made with essential oils and marketed as natural or aromatherapy products.

Aromatherapy is based on the principle that certain scents will induce or encourage different feelings or emotional states: in which case, as I once overheard in a health-food shop, 'They should aerial spray the whole country with lavender so everybody can calm down.'

Perfumes can often cause an allergic reaction, particularly if worn in the sun, as this can cause chemicals to react differently with the skin. This is more common with citrus-based scents than others.

Perfume extract is usually 20 to 25 per cent perfume essence in 90 to 95 proof alcohol. *Eau de toilette* is 5 to 8 per cent essence diluted in 80 to 90 proof alcohol. The perfume may cost ten times as much but be only three times more concentrated. But you may use more *eau de toilette* to get the smell level up.

Have you ever been stuck in a lift or on a bus with somebody who uses too much perfume or aftershave? It's because they become immune to the strong smell, incorporating it into their senses without smelling it themselves. So they build up to putting more and more perfume on every day until the rest of us fall to the floor pleading for mercy, or at least some *air*.

A perfume's price takes into account the cost of ingredients, research and development, exclusivity, design, packaging, advertising, distribution, designer name and what people will be prepared to pay.

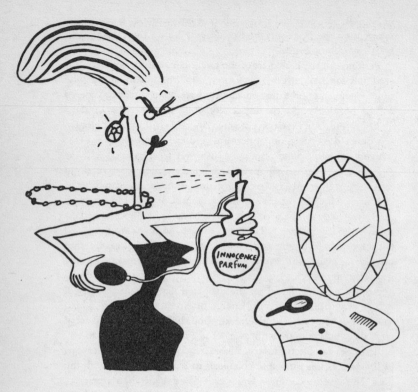

(Snobbery is the original aromatherapy.) Advertising campaigns now run into the millions for a single perfume.

Even perfumes that are not heavily advertised or that don't need a launch can chew through the bucks. According to one documentary, a £32 bottle of Chanel Number 5 perfume (which was the same cost per ounce as gold at the time) is worth about £1.50 in ingredients. The rest is money added by administration costs, packaging, advertising and profit.

Stinko bizarro Perfume must be one of the hardest things to sell. I already like it, but which to buy? All I want is a perfume that smells exactly like a fresh, trembling tuberose but what I get is pictures of Elizabeth Taylor looking as if she's totally lost her marbles, 11-year-old girls poncing around in evening gowns with velvet trains, women (who look as if they're struggling with an eating disorder as well as a dirty great bit of kelp) writhing at the water's edge, a young woman with feathers coming out of her bum wearing a leg leash, a man lurking around with a bunch of peonies, pictures of one naked person giving another one a firefighter's lift, very many pictures of women looking wistfully air-headed surrounded by baskets of floristry and a whole lot of absolute crap written to describe a scent.

Magazines now carry perfume samples, and many American magazines carry up to three separate perfume samples as part of the full page advertising. (In America you don't need to buy perfume. You just slink up to a newsstand and rub yourself against page 57 of something.)

In Britain, they're squabbling over more than £140 million in sales of women's perfumes in department stores, plus nearly £160 million at chemists and £62 million in department stores for men's fragrances. So they spend up on their launches of new scents. The perfume companies have monstrously lavish cocktail parties, dinners and parties with fireworks and caviar and obsequious waiters and lots of alcohol and free samples. They invite their closest personal friends: the Press.

After all, advertisers are flogging a wee bit of luxury for the people who can't afford to get invited to the perfume launch parties with caviar and fireworks and *marvellous* old Oscar de la Thingie flown over from (gasp, swoon, stagger) Paris! A bit of romance and glamour in a beautiful bottle. And some of the bottles are very beautiful, delicate, mysterious, gloriously chunky, designed by surreal artists and marketing geniuses. Others push the point, with fake jewels and golden metal butterflies.

We're buying Diamonds and Rubies from Elizabeth Taylor, and Trésor (Treasure) and Tweed, Lace, White Satin and White Linen that we can't afford to buy or wear because we live in the real world where white linen is impractical. We're buying the sexy, the forbidden, the racy, Volupté, Poison, Tabu, Joy and Opium. We want to be Knowing, Clandestine, Spellbound, Unforgettable, Beautiful, a Diva, a Paradox; to have Worth, Youth Dew, Mystery and Panache. We want to associate with a lifestyle: be Miss Dior, be in Paris, or more specifically one of its suburbs, Rive Gauche, or smell of its old

money, called Chanel Number 5. We want it for Eternity, Forever.
Or at least until 4711.

There are no perfumes called Pre-Menstrual Bitchface or Sheer
Poverty.

Hair

It's compulsory Hair:
we're covered in it. Although
some of it is more luxurious,
some is short and curly, and
some grows all the time and has
to be cut to maintain its length.
Other bits don't grow long,
which is very handy under the
circumstances. I don't fancy an
armpit ponytail myself.

Everyone has hair on the
legs, arms, face and pubic area.
In fact, everyone has hair all
over the body. Some have more or darker hair which is more noticeable on paler skins. We all get hairier as we get older. If your hair feels
dead, it's because it is: all the stuff above the skin surface, anyway.
That's why you can't repair split ends by doing anything except cutting them off. Eating a balanced diet with protein will make the hair
a healthier corpse. Hair is made from keratin, which is a form of
protein. You can damage your hair with sun, bleach, heat treatments
and blow-drying, perms and chemical dyes. Crash diets and stress
can cause temporary hair loss until you correct the problem. (Hair loss
usually starts two to three months after your nutrition level drops.)

Hormonal changes at puberty and the menopause can make the
hair oilier. Women on the pill or who are pregnant report that some
perms simply won't take on their hair. Pregnant women have really
shiny hair. And when you go grey is haireditary.

Magazines regularly run stories about 'new hair products', some
claiming 'technological breakthroughs' in shampoo, conditioner,

My major problem would be hair: I have
more hair on my arms than my boyfriend.
I wax my upper lip and in between my
eyebrows and have since I was 13. My current boyfriend made remarks all the time
until I broke down and explained that you
just don't say those kinds of things to a
girl. There are some clothes I will not
wear, like bikinis, because I have a little
snail trail and a lower hairy back.

Lena, 19

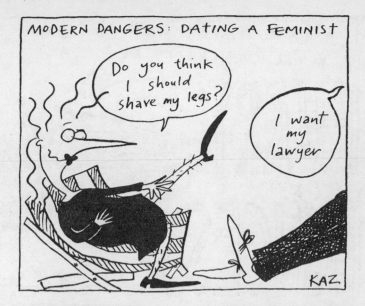

colour or removal. The last thing they want you to do is leave it alone and stop spending money on your furry bits. And remember, the more you do to your hair, the more you risk damaging it through heat, chemicals and harassment.

Getting it off An article in *Cosmopolitan* warbles on about 'reveal-it-all summer styles call for superbly smooth skin…Summer means lazy days at the beach and as most swimsuits are highcut and revealing, it's time to face that perennial hot weather problem: the abominable bikini line.' Or else it's time to face the fact that manufacturers are not producing enough swimsuits with low-cut legs that women want to wear.

Anyway, do you think this article on hair removal has anything to do with the fact that the next page is an ad for Johnson's baby oil and it says 'A Johnson and Johnson/*Cosmopolitan* promotion'? And then there's a page called 'A *Cosmopolitan* Andrea Promotion' and it's for

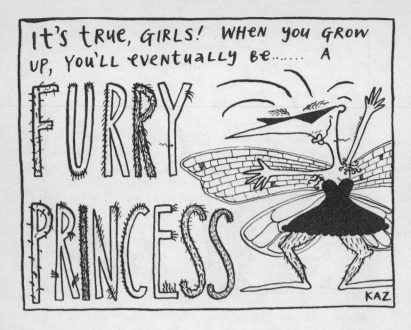

'Natural Wax Hair Remover'? What about the '*Dolly*/Waxeeze Promotion', in which what is basically an ad for hair-removal products is presented like a typical *Dolly* story with the magazine's layout and design style and a file photograph of a model with shorn legs? Let's get this straight. No magazine is likely to run a whole page of stuff on hair removal unless somebody is directly or indirectly paying for it.

I had my legs waxed for the first time as research for this book. Here are the results: it hurt like hell, my legs felt bald, startled and affronted, it cost about £20 and would 'have' to be done again in a few weeks (oh no, it wouldn't) *plus* it made my legs *itch* like crazy for several weeks afterwards.

Every 'expert' and doctor will tell you that hair does not grow back thicker and darker after it has been shaved, waxed or plucked but women say differently. Many people who fall into shaving away and rigorously plucking out most of their eyebrows, including models, have found that their eyebrows never grow back, or never the same way. Eyebrows are essential to the look of the face, which is why drawn-on false ones and plucked-practically-to-oblivion ones look so strange. They change the whole shape of the face and can give you a permanently quizzical, puzzled and witless expression. If you are determined to change your eyebrows, please don't shave them, not even once just a little bit. Plucking underneath is much less stressful than on the top of the brow. Whether you wax or pluck, it is going to hurt.

There are many ways women remove natural hair. There is shaving, which doesn't last long, waxing, which hurts, depilatory creams (virulent chemicals that dissolve the hair: spooky), electrolysis (in which a needle is poked into each hair follicle at the root of the hair and electrocutes the hair, which falls out and mostly does not grow back) which can leave permanent scarring if not done correctly and can also hurt and is meant to be permanent but sometimes has to be repeated several times on the same follicle, and plucking, which also hurts.

Drugs to make you less hairy can have truly horrifying side-effects and, in fact, are very, very rarely needed. Unless you have a history of abnormal menstruation or other symptoms of a hormonal disorder, the amount of hair you have is probably just your natural amount and nothing to do with a medical problem.

Whatever the fashion among your friends, hair removal is not compulsory.

PS: Try not to laugh if the person waxing your legs describes herself as an aesthetician.

Further help

If you're worried about a serious condition such as hair loss or major scalp flaking, the Institute of Trichologists will put you in touch with a trained trichologist. It would be safer not to trust a serious problem to a corner hairdresser. The Institute is at 228 Stockwell Road, London SW9 9SU. Phone 0171 733 2056. Send them a self-addressed, stamped envelope for a list of trichologists throughout the world, and further information on trichology.

When there's a society for the prevention of bossy hairdressers, I will let you know.

real *gorgeous*

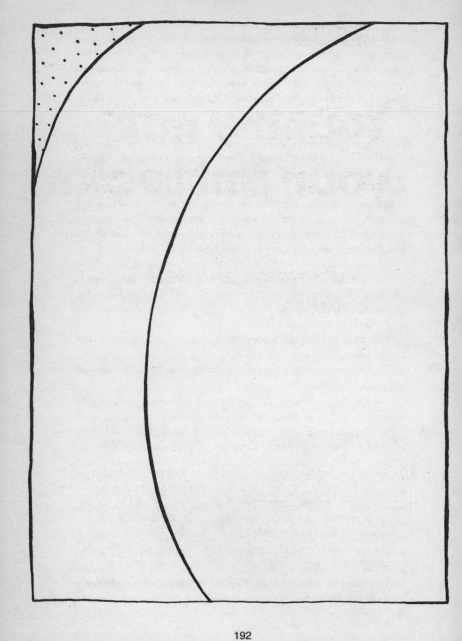

192

chapter *six*

You are not your buttocks

Self-image and self-esteem

Love the one you're with For a long time women's self-esteem has been tied to their feelings about physical appearance. Women are told not only that 'you are what you eat' but 'you are what you look like'.

With so much criticism, it can be hard to 'love the one you're with'.

Health workers have observed that eating behaviour and body image are closely connected. 'For women, this connection is deeply related to their self-esteem, as it seems they have always been valued as objects of beauty and desirability…however, this is somewhat different from men who obtain their self-esteem via achievements, power status and control,' according to a manual for health workers who are setting up body-image groups.

The manual says what is needed is social change, and 'educating women to explore their own body shape and what's comfortable and healthy for them, and alerting them to the social and economic forces so that they too can challenge them…it is about challenging women to value and see themselves as a whole person, and celebrate their body as both decorative and functional.'

The Body Image project identifies that a woman feeling unhappy or worthless will not express herself that way, but instead say, 'I'm fat' or 'I'm ugly'. This grossly distorted view has become 'normal' behaviour in women. Instead of decoding the feeling 'I am fat' to find that we are feeling unloved, dull or depressed, many of us just relate it to our body size or shape.

A university study found that in 35 surveyed couples, the women chose significantly thinner photographs to indicate

> I have panic attacks about being fat. When I look in the mirror I see a thin/skinny person, but as soon as I walk away I imagine myself as fat. I know what I'm doing, and I chastise myself for being ridiculous, but the paranoia is overwhelming.
>
> Graffiti in University law faculty women's toilets

what they thought their partners wanted than those their partners actually chose. Another study of 92 adults, 78 teenagers and 71 children showed that women and teenage girls – not men and teenage boys – believed they were larger than they needed to be to appear attractive.

Disturbingly, both the boys and girls aged nine and ten rated their figures as larger than ideal. The researchers concluded that 'one can only speculate that the imagery surrounding fatness and slimness as demonstrated on television and through other media is very influential in determining children's beliefs'.

Cleo magazine's dieting survey showed that 73 per cent of participants envied somebody else's body every day, and that every day more than half of the women felt depressed about their weight. Seventeen per cent avoided mirrors altogether. Others saw a distortion in the mirror.

≈♡≈

Pressure to have bad body image Where do we start? The censored image of women in TV and film shows only the thin; magazines suggest that body 'flaws' should be disguised, dieted against or exercised away. A Clarins ad (after writing this book I am beginning rather to despise the Clarins corporation) has the headline 'No body is perfect' next to a very thin, tall model with flawless (or airbrushed) skin. 'Get closer to the perfection you desire with Clarins plant extract-based treatments...You can concentrate on specific concerns like the bust or maybe you want a firmer derrière... Stubborn thighs, hips and bottoms...Lift and tighten...with the ultimate body control Clarins Body Shaping Gel'. Thighs, hips and bums are not 'stubborn' any more than they are 'confused' or 'happy'. Body parts do not have personalities or feelings.

The woman on the billboards in the lingerie ads is nearly one-quarter thinner again than the average woman, and much taller as well. Even if the model were of average height she could put on eight to ten more kilos without causing any health problems. But she is touted as having 'the perfect body'.

The definition of 'the perfect body', indeed, the idea that there might be only one, has been announced by media commentators who have no right to do so. There is more than one definition of a 'good body' or a 'fabulous body'. A 'perfect body' is a myth.

Body hatred is fashionable. Young girls watch adult women, and they know that one of the ways to be a big girl, a grown-up is that we have to grab hold of a part of ourselves with disgust and say, 'Look at this, I'm too fat.' Everyone else says, 'No you're not, I am. Look at this! Feel this!' grasping bits of themselves. Part of being a woman is projected as specific self-loathing in the face of evidence to the contrary. Anybody observing can see that the flesh being grabbed is not too fat.

> – How do you get a boyfriend?
> – Be yourself.
>
> My boyfriend was attracted to me because of my size. He loves huge buttocks and breasts and the confident way in which I walk...I hope you're as happy as I am.
>
> **Graffiti in Melbourne University women's toilets**

And still the self-definition insists: the distortion is lore, and law.

At only six and a half stone, 1960s model icon Twiggy said she 'hated what I looked like...I ate like a horse and just burned off everything. Like most skinny people, I desperately wanted to put on weight.' When very thin singer Margaret Urlich appeared on the Australian sports program *Live and Sweaty,* envious host Elle McFeast jokingly abused her for being thin, in the 'you're so thin, you bitch' tradition. Urlich stood up and twirled in mock triumph. Women who are thin are constantly referred to as 'lucky'. The rest of us, it is assumed, must work to become more like them.

Being thin Thin women are not immune from body hatred and bad self-image and esteem. Thin girls are taunted about being bony and skinny and not having prominent breasts. Nasty comments are made questioning their femininity, their warmth as human beings and whether they have an eating disorder. There are rude, envious comments: 'You're such a bitch, you're so thin.' One thin woman, writing of her experience in a newspaper, said, 'There are many garments the thin female shouldn't wear. Like clothes that expose just about any part of the body…not a pretty sight. Would the old chook who is exposing her horrible scrawny knees on the Melbourne cocktail party circuit please take note?…When you lose weight the first thing to go are the bosoms, of course …women tend to be flat-chested if their other vital statistics are pared down. Sexy isn't exactly the word for a Skinny Minnie at the beach or in her lingerie.' But thin woman are just as sexy as bigger ones, and no less womanly for having smaller curves.

> I spend a lot of time writing letters to readers, particularly the younger ones, repeating the phrase, 'If you are within the healthy weight range for your height and are fit, healthy and active, you have every right to be proud of your body'. I don't know how many take it to heart though. It's one of those things that's very easy to accept intellectually, but so hard to truly believe…I also find myself writing to people (to tell them) they must put out of their heads the idea that by losing the weight they will automatically look like a fashion model. No amount of dieting is going to make a wide-hipped woman of 150 cm decrease the size of her pelvis and grow 30 cm (in height). It seems to me that…most of us think if we can get this right, every other aspect of our lives will automatically be perfect.
>
> Diane Parks,
> *Slimming* magazine

Just like everybody else In adolescence, the changes in our body are the first real major changes since we started walking and talking. Our families talk about the changes, and maybe they tease us. Kids at school notice development or no development. We want to shrink into the crowd, be like everybody else, too obsessed and freaked out to notice that everybody else is freaked out and different too. Even those who are teasing us. We read magazines to find out how to be 'normal', how to look like everybody else. This is exactly the way to become a dull or scared person: perhaps more likely to be picked on.

Self-esteem and puberty According to a study conduct-
ed by the Australian Institute of Sport, which mimics international findings, the self-confidence levels of boy and girl athletes at about age 13 and 14 are pretty much identical, and after that they drop off, but the female level drops off quicker and to a greater extent than the male level. The study adds, 'For both sexes it seems to bottom out or reach its lowest levels at around 19, 20, 21 years of age and then it bounces back out again, but interestingly the males actually end up higher than when they started, and the female athletes never reach the same level [as at 13 and 14] again.'

This research suggests that even the female 'winners' in our society – the study was of 1798 athletes over six years to 1989, who were physically fit and still winning – will reach a peak of self-esteem before puberty and never again reach that level as young people or adults.

Similar results were found by a 1991 study of 200 14 to 15 year old students called Adolescents' Problems and Their Relationship to Self-Esteem. Girls' self-esteem declined dramatically at puberty: girls were more concerned about societal and personal relations, courtship, sex, marriage and physical development. Boys were more concerned about finance, education and career issues.

> Throughout my early teens I did not like myself and thought I was chubby. I look back at photos of myself and see that I was actually quite slim: and in fact slimmer than some of the girls I envied.
>
> Carol, 19

The authors of the study said some things became clear from asking young people what they think: 'While the media promotes an image of the physical, personal and interpersonal attributes that girls should attain, it virtually ignores those areas for boys, who are encouraged to become educated, combative and aggressive for personal and economic survival.'

> Not even my academic achievements can drag me up out of the dumps when I am confronted with...The Mirror! I am confronted almost every day in the mirror at ballet class where the leotards and tights tell everyone about the chocolate I ate at lunch.
>
> Diana, 20

Educational research indicates that girls are inclined to explain their successes by external factors, such as help from parents and teachers and luck, but blame themselves for failures. Boys usually blame failure on bad luck or unfair tests. It seems we could learn something from the boys.

 Deborah Saltman, an associate professor of social and preventative medicine, says girls have a lot of trouble with their changing bodies, and can feel 'freakish'. They also have to come to terms with double standards about their sexuality – they should be sexy-looking, but also be 'good girls' without a bad reputation. Dr Saltman says girls need to know that adolescence is a time of big changes, where you can experiment, make mistakes, and feel whatever it is you're feeling – angry, sad, not like talking, whatever. (Of course, your family will probably think you are a drug addict.)

How to like yourself US psychologist Thomas Cash and graduate student John Buttershave created a body-image therapy which combines body education, relaxation techniques and guided imagery to change ingrained body-image distortions. Patients are taught to move from: 'I'm so ugly. Everyone looks better than me', to 'I like the way I look. I don't mind people looking at me'. Sometimes this takes months. One woman who did the course says she still thinks her thighs and hips are too big,

> One of the things I have that slightly cheers me up is a picture of Marilyn Monroe. She's trying on a black bikini and my God, she's absolutely fat and she looks wonderful.
>
> Kim, 23

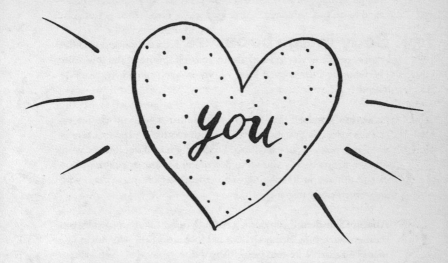

but she doesn't dwell on it and is able to go to beach parties.

Many women's health centres, hospitals and community centres run body-image courses. Body-image groups are usually small — six to eight people — and women only. They encourage participants to stop thinking about the body as parts of a machine that need to be controlled, and to think of the whole body. Participants keep a journal and study their inner voices to hear if that's them talking, or society, or somebody else. Attitude to food is also explored, including other experiences that can make you feel rewarded, and nutrition information. Participants learn that their body knows what shape and size it needs to be. You have to listen to what your body really needs: a decent feed and the odd bit of exercise.

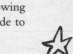

 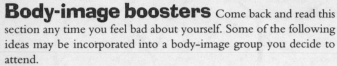

Body-image boosters Come back and read this

section any time you feel bad about yourself. Some of the following ideas may be incorporated into a body-image group you decide to attend.

Examine yourself Stand in front of a mirror with no clothes on (lock the door!). You can start with your clothes on the first time if you can't look at your nakedness. Describe yourself out loud or write it down neutrally, as if you were describing a statue or painting. You can do this as you are rubbing in a moisturising cream, perhaps with an aromatherapy fragrance.

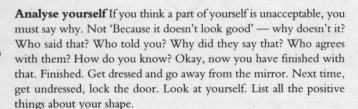

Analyse yourself If you think a part of yourself is unacceptable, you must say why. Not 'Because it doesn't look good' — why doesn't it? Who said that? Who told you? Why did they say that? Who agrees with them? How do you know? Okay, now you have finished with that. Finished. Get dressed and go away from the mirror. Next time, get undressed, lock the door. Look at yourself. List all the positive things about your shape.

Live happily in your body Some ways of feeling that your whole body is you and not just a whole lot of bits latched onto you like carpet fluff, include doing regular exercise such as swimming, walking or yoga. I know I always feel better about my body, lighter and more together after I do yoga. Yep, those three mornings a year I remember to do my yoga are always truly great. Other postural and movement disciplines, including the Alexander technique and dancing (*not* ballet or gym or anywhere else where they panic about their weight), can be useful. A young woman who took belly-dancing lessons in Melbourne said, 'Through the dance, my body expresses itself in ways I haven't heard before, the lumps and bumps get a chance to speak. It's like a body language. My legs are heavy for my size but in dance they are supportive'. The other girls and women from the class said dancing together had given them a more realistic image of women's bodies.

 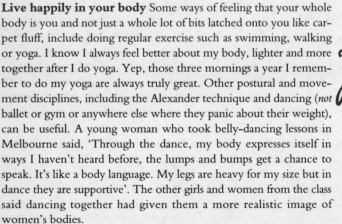

Exercise In general, fit and healthy people feel better about themselves. People who take care of themselves (thanks, but no more unprocessed whale lard for me and I don't think I will have that fourteenth pint of Guinness), can find they have a corresponding realisation that they are worth caring about. This is not the false 'caring about yourself' that involves things like depriving yourself of food and overexercising, or wearing make-up but not having that changing mole checked, or ironing your clothes but having sex without a condom.

Analyse messages Every time you see a magazine article telling you to be thinner, exercise more or wear more flattering clothes, don't let it hang like a personal accusation. Ask first: Why is the magazine running this story? To sell clothes, to sell cosmetics? Because they believe it? Because they're too scared to stop? Because they know we're all interested in body image and they know their story on it, positive or negative, will boost sales? Why should I listen to this? What will happen if I reject this idea? What will happen if I recycle this magazine and go and have a bar of chocolate?

Reward yourself Choose a variety of treats, not just food – bubble baths, girls' nights out, holidays, congratulations, a new book, red shoes, flowers, art, whatever takes your fancy.

Be realistic As the editor of American *Ms* magazine, Robin Morgan says about feminism, 'Change doesn't come from the top'. Don't expect the magazines to change; they will not, unless we force them. And even then, the advertiser's dollar will be stronger than ours. *Ms* magazine has no ads for this very reason – so its editorial content will not be influenced by advertising. It has no articles on hair, no weight-loss diets, no cosmetics, no fashion.

Describe yourself Penelope Goward, from the Body Image Project, says it is important for girls to stop seeing their physical selves as 'the most important aspect of their whole being'. So here's another exercise (and you don't have to do anything like a leg lift). Sit

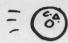

down somewhere quiet and make a list of all your attributes. Pretend you are describing yourself in minute detail to somebody from another planet you have never met, who will have to guess who you are. You are not allowed to refer to anything physical whatsoever. Make a list of all your positive characteristics and knowledge. Make a list of what your friends like about you. Try describing your friends without making reference to their appearance.

Be a whole person Achieve in other areas, gain control of other areas, so you don't get obsessed with the outside of yourself. This may mean joining a team sport, exploring an artistic pastime, developing an interest in film, photography, nature studies, politics, engineering. Join a rock band, write songs, draw cartoons, act, run, sew, cook, embrace experiences and chances, make jokes. Hang out with people who accept you and like to do things, who don't just sit around talking about bodies, diets, tanning and obsessing about food. That's boring and passive.

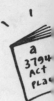

Get to know your body Learn anatomy, have massages, acupressure, foot reflexology. Feel yourself breathing, exercising, relaxing.

Fight the body police Prepare ways to respond to people who feel they can comment on and judge your appearance, even those who think they are being 'helpful'. (You will find some hints in the Body Police section.)

Clean house Throw away pictures of models you might have cut out or kept in your head that you have aspired to. Understand that they are *them* and you are *you.*

Accept your genes Look at different members of your family and family photographs as far back as you can go. Recognise family traits, without judging them as good or bad.

Be a pal When possible, support other women and girls in their

     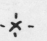

body image. I can still remember my aunt saying to me as a teenager, 'You have beautiful, strong legs. They're wonderful'. I was sceptical but she was obviously sincere, so I was forced to consider what she said. I can also remember a great-aunt saying rudely and dismissively in front of me, about me, but not to me, 'She's very *solid* isn't she?' I still love the first aunt, and I wouldn't give you 20 cents for the other one, who was a lot more solid than I was and probably felt better by insulting me. Maybe she didn't think at all, maybe she was just brainwashed.

Analyse your feelings Another suggestion from the Body Image project is to change the way you talk about yourself from negative to neutral or optimistic phrases. Write down the things you know you have said about yourself and look at other ways of expressing them. For example, 'My skin looks disgusting' could become 'I am freaked out about my skin'. 'I look worse than ever' may become 'I usually look better than I do now'. 'I hate my fat hips' translates to 'My hips are the widest part of me'.

Stand up for your rights Defend the gains women have made in being taken as individuals and recognised for their talents and contributions, not just for what they look like. Support equal opportunity at home and at work and preserve and celebrate the institutions, laws and people who are still fighting for that equality.

Be a really whole person See your body as your home, the kind thing you live with, in and as. Not as something separate from you.

Express yourself Put on a tape or the radio and sing. Loud. Really loud. Belt it out. When the neighbours come to complain, explain it's for your self-esteem. See if you can get them to dance. Singing is expressing yourself, an emotional release. Joining a drama group will also help boost self-esteem. If you feel overwhelmed by the awful inner voice telling you that you are too fat, get it out, in poems, drawings, songs, a diary or journal. Exercise it and may it be exorcised.

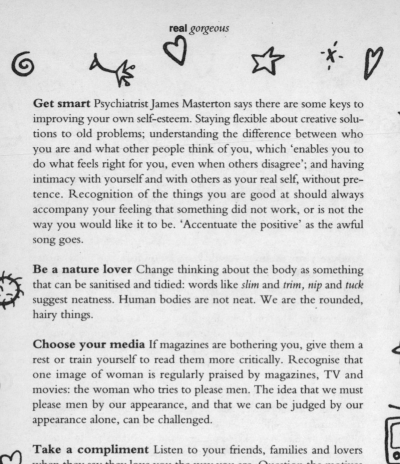

Get smart Psychiatrist James Masterton says there are some keys to improving your own self-esteem. Staying flexible about creative solutions to old problems; understanding the difference between who you are and what other people think of you, which 'enables you to do what feels right for you, even when others disagree'; and having intimacy with yourself and with others as your real self, without pretence. Recognition of the things you are good at should always accompany your feeling that something did not work, or is not the way you would like it to be. 'Accentuate the positive' as the awful song goes.

Be a nature lover Change thinking about the body as something that can be sanitised and tidied: words like *slim* and *trim*, *nip* and *tuck* suggest neatness. Human bodies are not neat. We are the rounded, hairy things.

Choose your media If magazines are bothering you, give them a rest or train yourself to read them more critically. Recognise that one image of woman is regularly praised by magazines, TV and movies: the woman who tries to please men. The idea that we must please men by our appearance, and that we can be judged by our appearance alone, can be challenged.

Take a compliment Listen to your friends, families and lovers when they say they love you the way you are. Question the motives of those who don't and plot ways of getting away from their undermining.

Give compliments But ask yourself what kind of compliment you are giving. Are you telling somebody by your actions or conversation that you think they are interesting, worthy, healthy-looking, happier, with a fabulous new pair of shoes? Or are you saying 'You look good because you look thinner': a much more boring and ultimately destructive compliment that says more about your own problems with shapes and sizes than what you think of the other person.

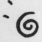
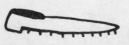

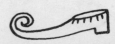

How to find a body-image group

Ask at your local community or women's health centre, the regional health authority, local hospital, or eating disorders support group for one to join, or start one with their help.

Further reading

Dr Judith Rodin, *Body Traps* (Arrow Books, 1993)

Starhawk, *Truth or Dare Encounters with Power, Authority and Mystery* (Harper and Row, San Francisco, 1987). Discusses issues of power and body image.

Kim Chernin, *Womansize: The Tyranny of Slenderness* (Women's Press, London, 1983)

Dr Marcia Hutchinson, *Transforming Body Image* (The Crossing Press, Freedom, California, 1985)

The body police

Hassled by the body police Families, relatives and friends feel they have a right to comment on a girl's body when it begins to change at puberty. Girls are taught to expect exposure and commentary and judgement from others, often based on unrealistic ideals. The girls are shamed and turn to dieting and exercise. Penelope Goward, head of a Body Image project, also notes this. 'If you have received negative feedback about your body as a child and adolescent, you will have low self-esteem about your body when you grow up.'

How to deal with the body police So many of the girls

real *gorgeous*

I loathed mirrors and shopping for clothes. When I was 16 something changed. I discovered the world of performing arts...I left my school to go to a performing arts course in Year 12. My folks were horrified. They said I could not succeed because I was 'fat'. But I wasn't doing it as a career move, I was doing it to gain confidence in myself. And I did gain confidence, slowly. According to conventional tables I am 40 kilos overweight. I've always had plenty of boyfriends and offers for as long as I have felt confident about myself. I have recently started working as a photographic model and a life-drawing model: confident women of my shape and size are in short supply so I'm getting plenty of work. I still have my 'fat days', my 'ugly days' and my 'bad hair days' but I am generally satisfied with the way I look.

Willa, 24

I hate being skinny. When I get sick I have no reserves and feel so weak and skinny: it's a really scary feeling. I believe there is too much pressure on females to look great. What is inside is much more important. I am finally learning this. Someone who is only average-looking can appear so beautiful – if they are happy and kind on the inside it will make them glow with beauty on the outside.

Mandy, 21

I hate my face because it's too fat. I would much rather be anorexic than obese or overweight. When I look in magazines I think how I'd love to be skinny. Everywhere I look there are skinny people, which makes me hate myself even more. I have tried to commit suicide about four times. I wish magazines would stop portraying 'fat' as being bad.

Amy, 16

and women who wrote to me about this book, responding to a request printed by *Cleo* and *Dolly* magazines, could remember the comment that first started them dieting, and often spurred them on to an eating disorder, especially bulimia.

Perhaps if you show this book to members of your family they will realise the damage their 'joking' or judgement may have. Explain to them they might have forgotten that the natural changes at puberty don't match the pictures of girls and women seen in magazines and on TV. Let them know that their comments – about something you cannot and should not try to control – are training you for food obsessions, eating disorders and a lifetime of self-loathing. Ask them to accept you the way you are.

If they don't, try to remember that so many parents, especially

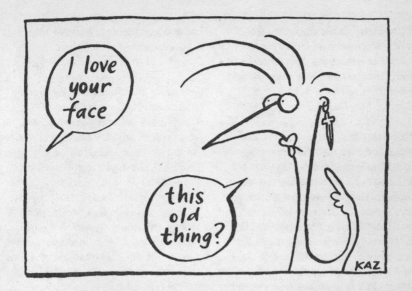

mothers, have been subjected to the same nasty pressure about bodies and the fear of fat. They can project their fears on to you through comments such as 'You're getting fat', even when you are a perfect shape and size for yourself. (Remember that you may have different genes than your mother or sisters.)

You can use this book to show your family that dieting does not work, and that if you eat healthy foods and exercise three times a

At 5ft 6 tall, weighing around eight and a half stone, it hasn't been any easier for me to get dates or a boyfriend, wear clothes that I'd like to, meet more people, wear a bikini with confidence or anything else that 'fat' people think we do with ease. What it takes is confidence – confidence to love your body and love who you are.

Amanda, 17

I walked along the beach in the moonlight, looking down at my strong, rounded white legs. I suddenly thought, 'I like those legs. They're a bit strangely shaped and wobbly up the top, and they've got me around for 30 years, and dammit, I like them.'

Lucy

My boyfriend is only one or two stone heavier than me, but I feel larger than he is. He is also taller. My clothes can be literally falling off me (I am a size 10) and I still feel big and fat.

Annette, 25

Three years ago I put on a little bit of weight and went up to 66 kilos, which is okay. I was informed by my grandparents, sister and parents that I was 'getting fat'. I then changed to a gluten- and dairy product- free diet and exercised like mad. I lost 12 kilos. I was then told I'd lost too much weight. I've been called ugly, beautiful and pretty, hassled due to my big breasts and hips, called fat, skinny and a rake. What am I supposed to think? The main influence on me in these areas is my family. I am doing nursing and we are educated about positive self- esteem, eating disorders, weight ranges. But somehow, I don't know why, the experts and print media, although (probably) they give more truthful information, do not have the same amount of influence as those we know and the visual media.

Kathleen

One of the marching girls chaperones exclaimed, 'My God you're never going to fit into your uniform, I've never seen anyone grow outward so fast that much'. All the girls started calling me 'Big Mumma'. The tears came to swell in my eyes. Then I decided to only have dinner and starve myself all day and this went on for about a month. I became very moody, pale and very, very thin. The coach told my mum, she was very concerned but didn't do much about it. One morning I had an aching back. I had a look at it in the mirror and there were bruises all up my spine. I told my coach about it and she said it was the first sign of anorexia. I am now back on my feet and am 165 cm tall and 53 kilos and slowly recovering.

Tanya, 16

week for more than half an hour, you are the right size and shape for you. Many people will be surprised at this information because of the diets and propaganda they see in television and magazines and their own history of struggle with body image. They may not believe you because it is too confronting for them.

As for guys, the young ones who try to torture you with insults and comments are just absolute dickbrains. They are just trying to make themselves feel tougher. How many of them say these things when they are on their own? They don't have the guts or the reason: they have only been trying to impress their mates.

Girls and women who make cruel or thoughtless comments have the same motivation. If they can impress their standards on you, they can feel better about the dieting crap they put themselves through. If they see you are happy with what you are, they feel threatened because they are still trapped by the lies they have been told. They make themselves feel prettier and better by knocking you.

Older guys who still put pressure on women about their figures are ignorant. If you are with a man who puts you down for who or what you are, you are with the wrong man. If you continue to allow him to dictate your self-esteem, you will spiral down. You may end up being an emotionally or physically abused person, too cowed to know how to get away and find people who will appreciate you for yourself, and men who will think you're

Sure it's fine to please friends and family, but remember you only have one life and you should give yours a little bit more attention...If people do not like what you do or the way you look, it would be the person's problem, not yours. We have to start to realise that there is nothing wrong with ourselves individually and that only people who want to see faults and pick them out are the ones with the abnormality in society. Trying to be accepted by them...robs us of the opportunity of being unique and different to one another. It stops us from who we really want to be and feel comfortable being.

Penny, 17

'I'm skinny. Are you jealous?'
'Not at all. I am cuddly and soft. Are you jealous?'
'I'm fat and I have a great sex life.'

Graffiti in university
women's toilets

Throughout primary school and Years 1 and 2 I was the butt of some of the kids' jokes. I had and still have the 'big nose syndrome'. I would get the teasing, the name calling. It was terribly, terribly hard to ignore. When I got to Years 3 and 4 it ceased, almost. Still there are the totally obnoxious people at parties, that 90 per cent of the other people would love to impale on a sharp stick and set fire to. Although I am still very conscious of the bit of me that's unfairly dominant, I have a groovy time.

Irina, 18

'From now on you will not be having cakes or dessert,' announced my megalomaniac mother in front of the whole family. I was seven years old, for crying out loud. So I was put on the right track for a lifetime of eating disorders and self-image distortions. By the age of 11 I had reached my adult height. 'You could be so good looking if you weren't so fat. Fat people are ugly. Fat people are psychologically disturbed. Fat people don't get jobs because normal people don't trust them because they think they are greedy. I'm only telling you this because I care about you and I want to protect you from how other people will react. Don't look at cookbooks it will give you bad ideas.' I can't believe all of the abuse my parents put me through has had such a lasting effect.

Anonymous, 24

My friend says, 'My mum's never happy with me and tells me I need to go on a diet, but it's easy this way (bulimia)'. I had just bought a new outfit. All my friends commented on how great it looked on me and I thought so, too. I couldn't wait to get home and show Mum. To my disappointment this is what my mother said, 'Oh it looks great...although you just have to lose weight in your legs first, hey?' Most of my friends just want to please mum and get her approval.

Daisy, 17

I grew up in dancing classes from the age of three and have seen candid close-ups of the pain that girls and women experience when subjected to constant scrutiny about their bodies.

Julie, 20

gorgeous because they like you. They *are* out there but you won't find them if you stay in situations that reinforce bad feelings about yourself. If he doesn't shape up, ship out. He has the problem, not you.

When you cannot make your family understand, and when the comments come from people at school, at parties or in the workplace, you may need some help in dealing with the body police. Surround yourself as much as you can with activities and people who celebrate who you are and what you can do. Practise the self-esteem and body image boosters. Remember that one day you will be able to escape your family. If things get desperate, we may have to institute a helicopter rescue service.

My best friend started seeing a man who told me on a number of occasions I was overweight and should lose it. I became very self-conscious and went to see a dietitian. By eating sensibly and exercising three times a week I lost around nine kilos and others said I looked really good. Soon I was eating less and exercising six times a week. I was underweight but could not stop. I weighed myself every morning and thought about being fat at least every five minutes...I was admitted to an eating disorders unit. I was happier fat, but I just can't let go of wanting to be thin and accepted.

Cheryl, 23

If I ever went to my friend Karen's house she and her mother were trying to convince me to do the same as Karen and go on a diet.

Danni, 17

My brother is 15 years old and constantly makes remarks about my figure. If we are having a fight he calls me 'thunderthighs' or tells me to lose weight. I play netball, touch football and walk absolutely everywhere I can. At one stage 18 months ago I became very self-conscious about my body and began to vomit up my food. One day I was walking to the train station when a group of about six guys walked past me. One said, 'Fat legs baby,' and another said, 'Big arse'. I felt so embarrassed, humiliated but most of all, angry...Who do they think they are and how dare they say that to me, a total stranger? I see the same things happen in nightclubs – not just to me but to other girls with perfectly normal figures.

Allie, 18

I wish I could weigh more and have tried without success. I have a very small bust which I really wish I could change. During high school this worried me the most. I did get teased about this on a few occasions by guys mostly. I still get a little depressed when you see perfectly shaped women on television and in movies and when you hear a guy say something like the first thing that they look at when they meet a girl is her breasts or that they would only go out with a girl with big breasts.

Anonymous, 21

Things to say to the body police

Sometimes ignoring them will help, sometimes it encourages further abuse. Try not to fall into the trap of always returning an insult, as you can just get into a slanging match that teaches them nothing and drives you crazy. Sometimes, however, it might be the only way to drive home your point. Enlist your friends so you can help each other go on the offensive.

Ask yourself not, 'What can I do to make myself more acceptable?' but, 'What is the matter with that person that they need to judge me by their own insecurities and standards?' People who are truly happy with themselves never bother to slag off other people. There is always a reason why you are being targeted, and it has nothing to do with you.

Some of these suggested retorts (below) can be used as all-purpose responses to any body commentary from someone else, such as, 'Are you feeling insecure?', 'You wouldn't say that without all your mates around you', and 'Grow up!'

If you just don't feel safe saying any of these things out loud, make sure you say them to yourself. This can be most satisfying. Laughing or smiling after people insult you can drive them crazy. It's a great way to show you don't take their uninformed judgment seriously.

THEY say:
'You're getting a bit fat' (or disapprovingly, 'You're putting on weight').

YOU say:
'No, I'm not, I'm just growing.'
'No I'm not. What did you say that for?'
'Who asked you?'
'Why are you trying to upset me?'
'What is it you are feeling insecure about?'
'I am not fat, I'm me-shaped.'
'I'm growing. Any objections?'
'Anything else? Perhaps you could write it down for me so I don't forget?'

'How kind of you to say so.'

'I have no intention of going on a stupid, impossible diet just so you feel that your outdated prejudices are validated by pressuring me into action which would be counter-productive and unhealthy, thereby reinforcing the self-loathing recommended by you and your own fears. So, hey, get a life, dickbrain.'

'And you're a real heart-throb.'

'A bit fat for you, or a bit fat for me?'

'Why don't you grab your bottom lip and pull it over your head?'

'You have no right to comment on my body.'

'Yes, thank you, I have put on weight, and I feel great.'

'Thank you.'

'I'm not worried about it, so relax.'

'I'm sorry, but I don't care what you think.'

'Nobody was ever thrown out of bed for being cuddly.'

'When I need your opinion to make me feel crappy, I'll let you know.'

'You're right. I guess I should become anorexic immediately. Would that be all right?'

'Are you trying to give me an eating disorder?'

'You can get a book from the library to explain what shape women are.'

'What makes you so interested in my shape?'

'I'm not getting fat, I'm growing. It's this inevitable thing that happens when you're a teenager, like people hassling you.'

'You are quite right. I do not have the body of a 12-year-old boy. Do you have one you're not using?'

'What is this? Body insult hour?'

THEY say:
'Why don't you try the new diet/my new diet/a diet?'

YOU say:
'This is my natural shape. If it offends you, please don't look at it.'

'I don't need a diet. I eat healthy food.'

'Diets don't work.'

'I enjoy my food.'

'Because I'm not stupid. I know diets don't work.'

'Why don't you mind your own body?'

'This is really boring. Can't we talk about something else?'

'I don't want to get obsessed with food.'

'I'm happy the way I am.'

'Why do you want to run my life?'

'Why do you want to ruin my life?'

'Allow me to get away from you.'

'What makes you so interested in my body?'

'Strangely enough, I don't have time to go to the gym for five hours a day. Will I be arrested?'

'What's your problem?'

'Do I look that stupid?'

THEY say:
'You're a real skinny stick, aren't you? Have you got anorexia?'

YOU say:
'Is it my turn to criticise your body now?' 'No.'

'Who asked you?'

'Is there anything else you'd like to comment on? Should I take notes?'

'Thanks for that, Einstein.'

'Cat got your brain?'

'I am naturally thin. You, know, like you're naturally rude.'

'You mean I'm *thin*? Oh my God, I'd never noticed!'

'Small, but perfectly formed.'

'Good things come in small packages.'

'I am not a stick. I am a woman, with feelings.'

'Why don't you toss me over there and see if the dog fetches me?'

THEY say:
'You've got no tits.'

YOU say:
'Well, they're bigger than your brain.'

'Your fly is undone.'
'What's up your nose?'
'How long have you been looking at me?'
'That's not what you said last night in bed.'
'Feeling insecure?'
'Am I supposed to care what you think?'
'What makes you interested in my breasts?'
'Thank you for your intellectual contribution.'
'Dang, I knew I forgot something when I got dressed this
    morning.'
'Get a life.'
'You sound like a three-year-old.'

THEY say:
**'Cor, check out the big hooters on that' or 'Show us your
    tits'.**

YOU say:
'Show us your brain.'
Anything in a language they don't understand.
'Don't you know what they look like?'
'Grow up.'
'You can always tell a bottle-fed baby.'
'There's a big bogey coming out of your nose.'
'Never mind, when you grow up, a girl might show you
    what breasts look like.'
'Why are you so interested in my breasts?'

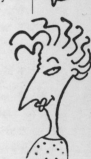

*An assertiveness training teacher tells me that this is a good method of pre-
    serving dignity and (we hope) making people realise how stupid they
    are being. Follow these five simple steps: stand or sit up straight. Pause
    for at least three seconds. Make firm eye contact. Use a well-modulat-
    ed voice to ask your question or make your statement. For example,*
'You're getting fat'. (Pause.) 'Am I?'
Or
'Aren't you too thin?' (Pause.) 'No.'

The Body Police Quiz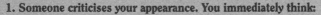

1. Someone criticises your appearance. You immediately think:

(a) I wonder what they're insecure about?

(b) Right that's it, I'm going to have my head removed.

(c) You might have left the iron on.

2. A guy in the street yells out: 'Hey, big arse!' You say:

(a) Excuse me, I think you might have dropped your IQ.

(b) Is that an eel coming out of your nose?

(c) What an attractive human being. That's the sort of man I really admire and like to be around. How about a date?

3. Your mother tells you you should lose some weight. You reply:

(a) Shall I amputate a leg?

(b) I'll start starving myself for your sake, shall I?

(c) Mum, I think you should read this stuff about why diets don't work.

4. Your family has been getting at you to lose weight. You call a family meeting and say:

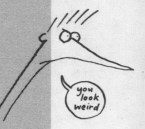

(a) We've got three choices. You stop hassling me, I get bulimia or you pay for me to go and live in the Bahamas. What'll it be?

(b) This is the shape I am. Your constant nagging does not take account of the fact that diets do not work, I am supposed to look like this, and you're driving me into becoming a neurotic, obsessed, miserable person. I just want to check with you if that's the whole point of this, in which case I am putting in an application to join another family. The Simpsons appeal.

(c) Either you accept me the way I am or I'm going to make extra pocket money by conducting guided tours of the lounge room of a dysfunctional family.

5. An uncle tells you you have started getting fat. You:

(a) Ask what it has to do with him.

(b) Tell him you could lend him a book on biology which would explain.

(c) Laugh at him.

6. A friend asks you to go on a diet with her. You reply:

(a) Only if it has KitKats, broccoli, turnips and custard in it.

(b) Thanks, but I can get bored at the same rate by watching paint dry.

(c) I'll race you to 15 kilos and the first one there's dead, nyah nyah nyah. Oh.

7. A girlfriend says, 'I'm so fat. I can't have lunch.' You react by:

(a) Explaining that if she doesn't have lunch she'll be inhaling chocolate by 3 pm.

(b) Saying 'You are not fat. That's flesh. It's for holding your bones in'.

(c) Who told you that? Come, we shall firebomb them.

8. You have always remembered the guy at school who said your nose is too big. You take comfort from the fact that:

(a) The guy is now living alone in a caravan with a part-time job as a sewerage sorter.

(b) He was only saying it to impress his mates, who collectively are as attractive to you as a four-hour documentary on the mating frenzy of toads.

(c) You have now moved on to a world unpopulated by smelly, 14-year-old boys who have the social skills of a ferret on drugs. He has asked you out three times.

chapter *seven*

In short

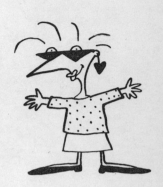

There are millions of gorgeous body shapes.
Yours is one of them.
Dieting doesn't work.
Your thighs are pretty cute.
Exercise should be fun not duty.
Expensive cosmetics may not be better than cheapies.
Advertising lies.
Plastic surgery sucks.
Modelling can be miserable.
You can recover from an eating disorder.
You can read magazines and watch television critically.
You can fight the body police.
You are not your buttocks.

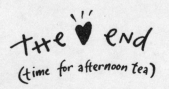

the ♥ end
(time for afternoon tea)

Contacts

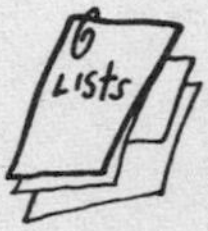

Women's Information and Referral Centres

For general advice on services available to women and referral to appropriate organisations.

Health

Eating Disorders Association
11 Priory Road
High Wycombe HP13 6SI
01494-21431
01603-621414

London Women's Therapy
Network
3 Carysfort Road
London N16 9AA
0171-249 7864 (North London)
0181-855 2510 (South London)

National Association for Mental
Health (MIND)
22 Harley Street
London W1N 1AP
0171-637 0741
Helpline: 0181-519 2122

SANELINE (information and
support for carers, sufferers and
friends) 0171-724 8000

Smokers Quitline
0171–487 3000

Women's Health
52-54 Featherstone Street
London EC1 8RT
0171-251 6580

Women's Health Concern
83 Earls Court Road
London W8 6EF
0171-938 3932

Women's National Commission
Caxton House
Tothill Street
London SW1 9NF
0171-247 5486

Natural Therapies

Traditional herbal medicine is being revived and expanded and is used to help people whom 'modern' medicine has failed, or who combine 'modern' medicine and natural remedies.

The most common ailments treated by natural therapists include reproductive and menstrual problems, fatigue, the immune system and recurring conditions (such as thrush), many chronic respiratory conditions and digestive disorders, including irritable bowel syndrome.

All natural therapists, including practitioners of traditional Chinese medicine, homoeopaths, naturopaths and herbalists, work with the body as a whole and have an emphasis on prevention.

Beware of the rare sort of hippy-dippy, so-called natural therapists who might claim that a decent dose of pollen juice will make an amputated leg grow back. You can check that your practitioner is accredited with a reputable organisation:

British Acupuncture Association
34 Alderney Street
London SW1V 4EU
0171-834 1012

British Holistic Medical
Association
179 Gloucester Place
London NW1 6DX
0171-262 5299

Institute for Complementary
Medicine
21 Poland Place
London W1N 3AF
0171-636 9453

Natural Institute of Medical
Herbalists
9 Palace Gate
Exeter EX1 1JA
01392-462022

Natural Medicines Society
Edith Lewis House
Ilkeston
Derbyshire DE7 8EJ
01602-329454

Register of Traditional Chinese
Medicine
7a Thorndean Street
London SW18 4HE
0181-947 1879

Yoga for Health Foundation
Ickwell Bury
Biggleswade
Bedforshire SG18 9EF
0176-727271

Northern Institute of Massage
100 Waterloo Road
Blackpool
Lancashire FY4 1AW
01253-403548

British Homeopathic
Association
27a Devonshire Street
London W1N 1RJ
0171-935 2163

British Chiropractic
Association
5 First Avenue
Chelmsford
Essex CM1 1RX
01245-358487

General Council and Register
of Osteopaths
1-4 Suffolk Street
London SW1Y 4HG
0171-839 2060

International Federation of
Aromatherapists
46 Dalkeish Road
West Dulwich
London SE21 8LS
0181-670 5011

Further reading

Ted Kaptuch, *Chinese Medicine: The Web That Has No Weaver* (Century, London, 1987)

Dr Stephen Davies and Alan Stewart, *Nutritional Medicine* (Pan Books, 1987)

Sporting Bodies

For advice on opportunities in sport access and facilities.

Sports Council
16 Upper Woburn Place
London WC1H OQP
0171-388 1277

Women's Sports Foundation
London Women's Centre
Wesley House
4 Wild Court
London WC2B 5AU
0171-831 7863

Human Rights and Equal Opportunities

Legal Action for Women
(LAW)
Kings Cross Women's Centre
71 Tonbridge Street
London WC1H 9DZ
0171-837 4509

National Alliance of Women's
Organisations
279-281 Whitechapel Road
London E1 1BY
0171-247 7052

Equal Opportunities
Commission (Press Office)
Swan House
52 Poland Street
London W1V 3DF
0171-287 3953

Head Office:
Overseas House
Quay Street
Manchester M3 3HN

Scotland:
Stock Exchange House
7 Nelson Mandela Place
Glasgow G2 1QW

Wales:
Caerwys House
Windsor Lane
Cardiff CF1 1LB

Northern Ireland:
Chambers of Commerce House
22 Great Victoria Street
Belfast BT2 7BA

Liberty – National Council for
Civil Liberties
21 Tabbard Street
London SE1 4LA
0171-403 3888

Commission for Racial Equality
Elliott House
10-12 Allington Street
London SW1E
0171-828 7022

Campaign for Freedom of
Information
88 Old Street
London EC1V
0171-253 2445

Amnesty International – British
Section
99-119 Rosebery Avenue
London EC1R 4RE
0171-814 6200

Cancer Organisations

For information about breast self-examination, lumps and cancer and
how to find an appropriate support group.

Breast Awareness Information
Tape: 0171-729 4915
Cervical Screening Information
Tape: 0171-729 5061

Breast Cancer Care
15/19 Britten Street
London SW3 3TZ
0171-867 1103
Nationwide free line: 0500-245
345

Scotland:
9 Castle Terrace
Edinburgh EH1 2DP
0131-221 0407

Suite 2/8 65 Bath Street
Glasgow G2 2BX
0141-353 1050

Cancer Care Society
21 Zetland Road
Redland
Bristol BS6 7AH
0117-942 7419

CancerLink
17 Britannia Street
London WC1X 9JN

Cancer Information Service:
0171-833 2451
Asian language line: 0171-713
7867
MAC helpline for young people
affected by cancer: free on
0800-591028

Scotland:
9 Castle Terrace
Edinburgh EH1 2DP
0131-228 5557

Northern Ireland:
The Ulster Cancer Foundation
40-42 Eglantine Avenue
Belfast BT9 6DX
01232-663281
Helpline:01232-663439
(9.30am-12.30pm, Mon–Fri)

Wales:
Tenovus Cancer Information
Centre
142 Whitchurch Road
Cardiff CF4 3NA
01222-619846
Freephone helpline:
0800-526 527

Eire:
Irish Cancer Society
5 Northumberland Road
Dublin 4
00 353 1 668 1855
Helpline: 00 353 1 800 200 700

Women's National Cancer
Control Campaign
128 Curtain Road
London EC2A 3AR
Helpline Counselling: 0171-729
2229

Safe Sex & Family Planning Association Headquarters

You still need condoms if you're in love: condoms are not just for casual relationships or One Night Stands.

If you are having sex—even once—you can get pregnant. Condoms are the only contraception which will prevent pregnancy and also guard against sexually transmitted diseases.

Some places you can hide condoms so they won't fall out include where you hide your tampons; in a cassette tape cover or CD cover; in a small purse with a zip or fold over flap.

Here are some things you can say to get a guy to wear a condom:

I don't want to get pregnant
I can't take the Pill: it makes me nauseous
Please do it for me
You look lovely in a hat
If you don't wear a condom I won't do it with you.

Sexually transmitted diseases

One or both of you might be carrying diseases WITHOUT knowing, as the symptoms are not always obvious, and sometimes mostly happen inside you. Some of them are incurable, some may develop to infertility or cancer, but ALMOST ALL of them are easily cured if treated early.

A guy can be infected with something and never know he has it. In this way, diseases can be passed on silently, without anyone knowing. Some sexually transmitted diseases have 'silent' symptoms—for example no visible sores or warts, or a symptom that could be mistaken for flu or period pains. And if not treated, some diseases will make you infertile.

Common sexually transmitted diseases include chlamydia, the wart virus, herpes, HIV (the AIDS virus), syphilis, gonorrhoea, and some forms of hepatitis.

For advice on contraception, Pap smear tests, pregnancy and abortion contact the relevant Family Planning office in your area and get details of your local clinic:

British Pregnancy Advisory Service
Henley-in-Arden: 01564-793225

Family Planning Association
Margaret Pyke House
27-35 Mortimer Street
London W1N 7RJ
0171-636 7866

Scotland:
2 Claremont Place
Glasgow G3 7XR
0141-332 1216

Wales:
Grace Philips House
4 Museum Street
Cardiff CF1 3BG
01222-342766

Northern Ireland:
113 University Street
Belfast BT7 18P
01232-325488

Marie Stopes House
Clinic and General Enquiries
The Well Woman Centre
108 Whitfield Street
London W1P 6BE
0171-388 0662

Marie Stopes Clinic
10 Queens Square
Leeds LS2 8AJ
0113-244 0685

Marie Stopes Clinic
1 Police Street
Manchester MN2 7LQ
0161-832 4260

National Aids Helpline
(24 hour) free confidential help
and advice 0800-567123

Terence Higgins Trust Helpline
(HIV and AIDS information)
0171-242 1010

Alcohol and Drug Counselling Organisations

Contact details are given for sources of information and counselling and referral centres.

Alcoholics Anonymous
11 Redcliffe Gardens
London SW10
0171-352 3001

Narcotics Anonymous (NA)
UK Service Office
PO Box 1980
London N19 3LS
0171-272 9040

National Alcohol Helpline
Weddel House
7th floor
13-14 West Smithfield
London EC1A
0171-332 0202

Release (for legal advice on drugs)
388 Old Street
London EC1V 9LT
0171-729 5255 (admin/publications 10am-5pm)
0171-729 9904 (advice line 10am-6pm)
0171-729 5255 (overnight helpline)

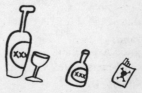

Counselling and Guidance Services

Carers National Association
Head Office
20-25 Glasshouse Yard
London EC1A 4JS
CarersLine: London: 0171-490
8898 (Mon–Fri, 1pm–4pm)

Childline
2nd Floor Royal Mall Building
Studd Street
London N1 0QW
0171-239 1000
Helpline: 0800 1111

The Compassionate Friends
(support for bereaved parents by
bereaved parents)
0171-953 9639

Cot Death Helpline (24 hour)
0171-235 1721

Cruse Bereavement Care
126 Sheen Road
Richmond TW9 1UR
0181-940 4818
Helpline: 0181-332 7227

Gamblers Anonymous
17/23 Blantyre Street
London SW10
0171-384 3040 (24 hour)

Gingerbread (provides lone parents with support and advice)
35 Wellington Street
London WC2E 7BN
0171-240 0953

Hysterectomy Support
Network
3 Lynne Close
Green Street Green
Orpington
Kent BR6 6BS

Institute of Family Therapy
43 New Cavendish Street
London W1M 7RG
0171-935 1651

London Lesbian and Gay
Switchboard (24 hour)
London: 0171-837 7324
and local switchboards

Message Home (left home?
Send a message, no questions
asked)
London: 0171-799 7662

The Miscarriage Association
01924-200799

Missing Persons Bureau
Helpline
0181-392 2000

National Council for One
Parent Families
255 Kentish Town Road
London NW5
0171-267 1361

Relate
0171-580 1087

The Salvation Army Family
Tracing Service
105 Judd Street
London WC1H 8EJ
0171-383 2772

Stillbirth & Neonatal Death
Society (SANDS)
28 Portland Place
London W1N 4DE
0171-436 5881

Students Nightline – National
Coordinators
c/1 Guild of Students
University of Birmingham
Edgbaston Park Road
Birmingham B15 2TU

Women's Environmental
Network
Aberdeen Studios
22 Highbury Grove
London N5 2EA
0171-354 8823

Emergency Counselling

You can ring and discuss your problem, at any time of the day or
night.

Rape Crisis Centre
0171-837 1600

Samaritans (24 hour)
0171-734 2800